Tarascon Medical Translation Pocketbook

From the publishers of the *Tarascon Pocket Pharmacopoeia*®

Ross I. Donaldson, MD, MPH
Assistant Clinical Professor of Medicine
David Geffen School of Medicine at UCLA
Director, Harbor-UCLA/IMC Global Health Fellowship
Department of Emergency Medicine
Harbor-UCLA Medical Center
Los Angeles, CA

Timothy Horeczko, MD
Clinical Instructor of Medicine
David Geffen School of Medicine at UCLA
Department of Emergency Medicine

JONES AND BARTLETT PUBLISHERS
Sudbury, Massachusetts
BOSTON   TORONTO   LONDON   SINGAPORE

World Headquarters
Jones and Bartlett Publishers
40 Tall Pine Drive
Sudbury, MA 01776
978-443-5000
info@jbpub.com
www.jbpub.com

Jones and Bartlett Publishers
Canada
6339 Ormindale Way
Mississauga, Ontario L5V 1J2
Canada

Jones and Bartlett Publishers
International
Barb House, Barb Mews
London W6 7PA
United Kingdom

Jones and Bartlett's books and products are available through most bookstores and online booksellers. To contact Jones and Bartlett Publishers directly, call 800-832-0034, fax 978-443-8000, or visit our website www.jbpub.com.

Substantial discounts on bulk quantities of Jones and Bartlett's publications are available to corporations, professional associations, and other qualified organizations. For details and specific discount information, contact the special sales department at Jones and Bartlett via the above contact information or send an email to specialsales@jbpub.com.

Copyright © 2010 by Jones and Bartlett Publishers, LLC
Cover Image: © Image Asset Management/age fotostock.

All rights reserved. No part of the material protected by this copyright may be reproduced or utilized in any form, electronic or mechanical, including photocopying, recording, or by any information storage and retrieval system, without written permission from the copyright owner.

All efforts have been made to assure the accuracy of this handbook. However, the accuracy and completeness of information in the *Tarascon Medical Translation Pocketbook* cannot be guaranteed. This book may contain typographical errors and omissions. Its contents are to be used as a guide only; healthcare professionals should use sound clinical judgment and individualize therapy in each patient care situation. Patient interaction and communication is an art that requires clinical intuition, experience, and good judgment. Cultural, linguistic, and individual factors play a part both in the message given and received. This book is meant to serve as a 'field guide' only and is not a substitute for a well-trained medical interpreter. This book is sold without warranties of any kind, express or implied. The publisher, editors, authors, and reviewers, disclaim any liability, loss, or damage caused by the contents.

The authors, editor, and publisher have made every effort to provide accurate information. However, they are not responsible for errors, omissions, or for any outcomes related to the use of the contents of this book and take no responsibility for the use of the products and procedures described. Treatments and side effects described in this book may not be applicable to all people; likewise, some people may require a dose or experience a side effect that is not described herein. Drugs and medical devices are discussed that may have limited availability controlled by the Food and Drug Administration (FDA) for use only in a research study or clinical trial. Research, clinical practice, and government regulations often change the accepted standard in this field. When consideration is being given to use of any drug in the clinical setting, the healthcare provider or reader is responsible for determining FDA status of the drug, reading the package insert, and reviewing prescribing information for the most up-to-date recommendations on dose, precautions, and contraindications, and determining the appropriate usage for the product. This is especially important in the case of drugs that are new or seldom used.

To our Patients, may we always find the right words.

—R.D. and T.H.

To my Grandfather, Mykola Horeczko, for his love and dedication to Faith, family, education, and the world's languages.

To my Parents, Bohdan and Carolyn, for their love and encouragement. Without them I would be nothing.

—T.H.

Production Credits
Executive Publisher: Christopher Davis
Senior Acquisitions Editor: Nancy Anastasi Duffy
Senior Editorial Assistant: Jessica Acox
Associate Production Editor: Melissa Elmore
Senior Marketing Manager: Barb Bartoszek
V.P. Manufacturing and Inventory Control: Therese Connell
Composition: Maryland Composition
Cover Design: Kristin E. Parker
Printing and Binding: Cenveo
Cover Printing: Cenveo

ISBN-13: 978-0-7637-6680-1
6048
Printed in the United States of America
13 12 11 10 09   10 9 8 7 6 5 4 3 2 1

CONTENTS

INTRODUCTION	vi
HOW TO USE THIS BOOK	vii
LIST OF CONTRIBUTORS	viii
LIST OF REVIEWERS	ix
MAP PAGE	x
UNIVERSAL PRONUNCIATION GUIDE	xi
QUICK REFERENCE PAGES	xii
CHOOSE YOUR LANGUAGE	xii
WHAT COUNTRY ARE YOU FROM?	xiii
HELLO!	xiv
PAIN?	xv
PAIN SCALE	xvi
CHAPTER 1 ARABIC	1
CHAPTER 2 FARSI	21
CHAPTER 3 FRENCH	41
CHAPTER 4 GERMAN	61
CHAPTER 5 HINDI	81
CHAPTER 6 ITALIAN	101
CHAPTER 7 JAPANESE	121
CHAPTER 8 KOREAN	143
CHAPTER 9 MANDARIN	163
CHAPTER 10 POLISH	185
CHAPTER 11 PORTUGUESE	207
CHAPTER 12 RUSSIAN	227
CHAPTER 13 SPANISH	249
CHAPTER 14 TAGALOG	269
CHAPTER 15 THAI	289
CHAPTER 16 UKRAINIAN	309
CHAPTER 17 VIETNAMESE	331
RESOURCES	351

LANGUAGE CHAPTER SECTIONS

INTRODUCTION & REGISTRATION
BASICS
GENERAL
QUALITY
ASSOCIATED SYMPTOMS
TIME COURSE
CONTEXT
PAST MEDICAL HISTORY
SURGICAL HISTORY
SOCIAL HISTORY
SYSTEMS REVIEW
GENERAL
HEENT
EYE
CARDIAC
PULMONARY
GI
GU
PSYCH
NEURO
MISC
GYNECOLOGIC
OBSTETRIC
TRAUMA
PEDIATRIC
PHYSICAL EXAM/INSTRUCTION
REASSESSMENT
PATIENT WORDS
PROCEDURES & CONSENT
TESTS
END OF LIFE
DISCHARGE
MEDICAL PROBLEMS
BODY PARTS
NUMBERS

INTRODUCTION

The polyglots are here to let you in on a little secret: you *can* speak another language! In fact, you've already learned at least one foreign tongue already: medicine. Listen to all the words spoken by your colleagues—you didn't know most of them when you were a kid. If you need to fix a medical problem, you instinctively use every resource at your disposal. How can you approach your patient, who doesn't speak English, and not do the same thing?

Don't worry if you haven't formally studied your patient's particular language. This book is set up to help you learn practical phrases as you go. Pull it out, read away, and don't be shy. Your patients and their friends and family can help you as you go. The best teachers are right in front of you and they are almost always happy to help.

You don't need to memorize endless lists of vocabulary or grammatical details that continue to become more confusing. Instead, just start speaking and you will find that your patients provide an abundance of non-verbal prompts. Don't think of it as an academic test, think of it as a game of charades. Point, mime, and read this book together. You can begin to communicate with only a few words.

Courage and this handbook are all that you need to begin. The sight of blood doesn't bother you – why should saying a bunch of syllables aloud be scary? Don't worry about sounding silly, just start with "hello" and you will be surprised how far you can go. Even if you end up using a translator, knowing a few words of your patient's native language will change the dynamics of your encounter. Patients are always grateful when you take time to get to know them better. You will be amazed at how many new doors will open as you use this book.

Ross I. Donaldson, MD, MPH
Chief Editor

Timothy Horeczko, MD
Senior Editor

HOW TO USE THIS BOOK

First, use the **Map** to help find out which language your patient speaks. Then, turn to the relevant language chapter **(see Contents)** for your particular patient.

Each language chapter contains commonly used medical phrases in the left column, followed by the phrases translated into the native language in the middle column, and then written in our Universal Pronunciation Guide on the right **(see page xi)**. Take a moment to familiarize yourself with this Pronunciation Guide—it is consistent throughout the book, whether you are speaking Arabic or Vietnamese. An additional column is included in some chapters for those languages with commonly used student pronunciation systems.

If you have little or no knowledge of the particular language, start slowly with words from the initial "Introduction" section within the selected chapter. Each language chapter is set up in the order of the classic medical history (current complaint, past medical, surgical, etc.). This is followed by a head-to-toe systems review, and then phrases for the physical exam, procedures, and summary remarks. At the end of each language chapter is an appendix of common medical problems, body parts, and numbers.

Phrases are constructed to be answered in a 'yes' or 'no' format whenever possible. If patients reply too quickly or with too long of an answer, it is sometimes helpful to simply repeat the question until answered clearly as a 'yes' or 'no.' Some phrases are meant to be put together with others, which are indicated by a '...' in the phrase.

We have purposely set up this handbook to integrate non-verbal prompts. Don't be afraid to point, use gestures, or read the book together with your patient.

GOOD LUCK!

LIST OF CONTRIBUTORS

LANGUAGE	CONTRIBUTORS
Arabic—العَرَبية	Maria Koleilat, MPH DrPH Student, UCLA School of Public Health
Farsi (Persian)—نابز	Ebrahim Kohannim, BS, MD Los Angeles, CA Omid Kohannim, BS, MS-II Medical Student, David Geffen School of Medicine at UCLA
French—Français	Lyly Cao Minh Medical Student, David Geffen School of Medicine at UCLA
German—Deutsch	Patrick R. Ryan David Geffen School of Medicine at UCLA
Hindi—भाषा	Ambrisha Joshi, MD Resident, Department of Pediatrics, Children's Hospital, Los Angeles
Italian—Italiano	Mark D. Sugi, MS-I Medical Student, David Geffen School of Medicine at UCLA
Japanese—日本語	Shota Yamamoto Medical Student, David Geffen School of Medicine at UCLA
Korean—언어	Jumie Lee, CPNP-AC, MSN Nurse Practitioner, Department of Emergency Medicine, Harbor-UCLA Medical Center
Mandarin Chinese—国语 (國語)	Hubert B. Shih, BS, BA, MS-II Medical Student, David Geffen School of Medicine at UCLA
Polish—Polski	Catherine Vojtus, MD Department of Emergency Medicine, Harbor-UCLA Medical Center
Portuguese—Português	Katya R. Calvo, MD Department of Medicine, Harbor-UCLA Medical Center
Russian—Русский язык	Timothy Horeczko, MD Clinical Instructor, Department of Emergency Medicine, Harbor-UCLA Medical Center
Spanish—Español	Timothy Horeczko, MD Clinical Instructor, Department of Emergency Medicine, Harbor-UCLA Medical Center Ross Donaldson, MD, MPH Asst. Prof. of Medicine, Geffen School of Medicine at UCLA
Tagalog (Filipino)—Tagalog	Maria Creselda B. de Leon, MS-IV Medical Student, David Geffen School of Medicine at UCLA
Thai—ภาษาไทย	Pauline Funchain, MD Resident Physician, Department of Medicine, Harbor-UCLA Medical Center Chutipat Greene, MS Alhambra, CA
Ukrainian—Українська мова	Timothy Horeczko, MD Clinical Instructor, Department of Emergency Medicine, Harbor-UCLA Medical Center
Vietnamese—Tiếng Việt	Huynh L. Cao, BS, MS-IV David Geffen School of Medicine at UCLA

LIST OF REVIEWERS

LANGUAGE	REVIEWERS
Arabic—العَرَبِيَّة	Engy Tadros, MD David Geffen School of Medicine at UCLA
Farsi (Persian)—نابز	Neda Jafarian, BS, MS-IV Charles Drew University of Medicine & Science
French—Français	Carolyn Anne Horeczko San Pedro, California
German—Deutsch	Valerie Neuhauser, RN Department of Emergency Medicine, Santa Monica-UCLA Medical Center
Hindi—भाषा	Mausam R. Damani, BA, MS-III Medical Student, David Geffen School of Medicine at UCLA
Italian—Italiano	Gianluca Rizzo Italian Department, UCLA
Japanese—日本語	Amy Kaji, MD, PhD Assistant Clinical Professor, Dept. of EM, Harbor-UCLA Medical Center/David Geffen School of Medicine at UCLA
Korean—언어	Edward Lee, MS-II Medical Student, David Geffen School of Medicine at UCLA
Mandarin Chinese—国语 (國語)	Victoria M. Ho, BS, MS-II Medical Student, David Geffen School of Medicine at UCLA
Polish—Polski	Adam Bronisz, B.S., R.T. (R) Department of Radiology, Harbor-UCLA Medical Center
Portuguese—Português	Claudia Mazzei, RN, MSN, FNP-C Nurse Practitioner, Department of Medicine, Harbor-UCLA Medical Center
Russian—Русский язык	Yuliya Keenan, RN Department of Emergency Medicine, Santa Monica-UCLA Medical Center
Spanish—Español	Marilee Carballo, MS-IV Medical Student, David Geffen School of Medicine at UCLA
Tagalog (Filipino)—Tagalog	Marc L. Montecillo, MS-II Medical Student, Charles Drew University/David Geffen School of Medicine at UCLA
Thai—ภาษาไทย	Andrew P. Dhanasopon, MS-IV Medical Student, Geffen School of Medicine at UCLA
Ukrainian—Українська мова	Bohdan Horeczko, PE Los Angeles, CA
Vietnamese—Tiếng Việt	Lien Doan, MD David Geffen School of Medicine at UCLA

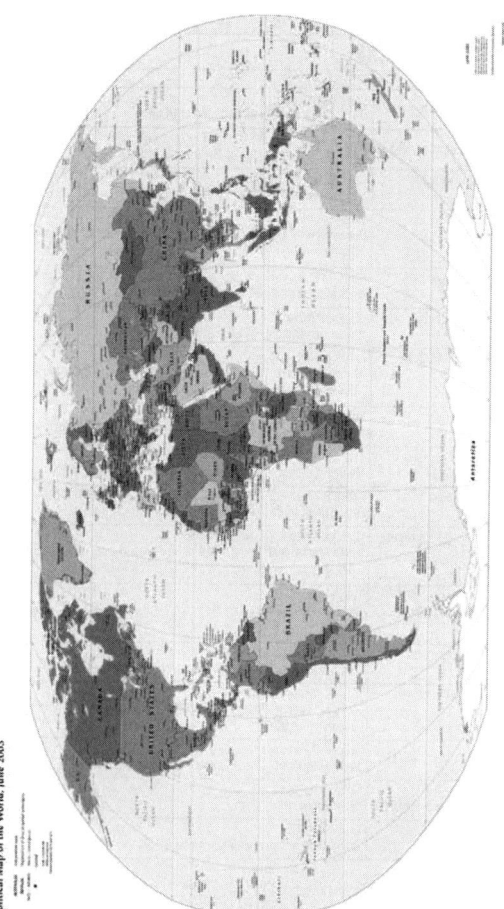

TABLE 1: UNIVERSAL PRONUNCIATION GUIDE

CONSONANTS		COMBOS	
B	*b*ut, we*b*	CH	*ch*air, tea*ch*
D	*d*o, li*d*	KH	lo*ch* (Scottish), Ba*ch*, *CH*ANUKAH
F	*f*un, enou*gh*, lea*f*	SH	*sh*e, *s*ure, lea*sh*
G	*g*o, *g*et, be*g*	ZH	plea*s*ure, bei*g*e
H	*h*am, *h*ouse	TH	*th*ing, *th*is
J	*g*in, *j*oy, e*dg*e	TS	i*ts*, ki*ts*, mi*ts*
K	*c*at, *k*ill, thi*ck*		
L	*l*eft, be*ll*	**FOREIGN**	
M	*m*an, ha*m*	RR	rolled "r" (i.e. as in Spanish)
N	*n*o, ti*n*	ng	nasalized: make the preceding vowel sound, but project the vowel from your nose, not from your mouth
P	*p*en, s*p*in, ti*p*		
R	*r*un, *r*abbit		
S	*s*ee, civil, pa*ss*		
T	*t*wo, s*t*ing, be*t*		
V	*v*oice, ha*v*e		
W	*w*ater, *wh*at	**DIPTHONGS**	
Z	*z*oo, ro*s*e	AY (A + EE)	m*y*, *eye*
VOWELS		AU (A + OO)	n*ow*, br*own*, c*ow*
A	f*a*ther, n*o*t, *au*ction	EY (E + EE)	d*ay*, h*ay*, m*ay*
E	b*e*d, l*e*t, m*e*t	YA (Y + A)	*ya*rd, *yaw*n
EE	s*ee*, b*ee*t, m*ee*t	YE (Y + E)	*ye*llow, *ye*s
O	n*o*, *oa*r, c*o*ld	YO (Y + O)	*yo*del, *yo*gurt
OO	s*oo*n, bl*ue*, sh*oe*	YOO (Y + OO)	*you*, p*u*pil, bea*u*tiful
I	c*i*ty, *i*t, f*i*t	YU (Y + U)	*you*ng, *yu*ck
æ	l*a*d, c*a*t, r*a*n	OY (O + EE)	b*oy*, k*oi*
U	r*u*n, f*u*n, p*u*t	WA (W + A)	*wa*ter, *wa*ll
		WE (W + E)	*we*ll, *whe*n, *we*t

Words are broken into syllables. "Capitalized words are stressed." (The English version of the preceding sentence would then be "KA-pi-tu-layz-d WOR-d-z ar STRES-d.")

Please note: Each language's sounds are only approximated by using the Guide; it is designed to give an English speaker the most authenticity possible, assuming no previous language experience.

Grammar: *m* = masculine form, *f* = feminine form.

TABLE 2: CHOOSE YOUR LANGUAGE

LANGUAGE	TRANSLATION	ENGLISH PRONUNCIATION
Arabic	العَرَبيّة	al a-ra-BEE-ya
Farsi	نابز	zæ-BAN
French	Français	f-kha-ng-SE
German	Deutsche Sprache	DOY-che SH-PRA-khe
Hindi	भाषा	ba-sau
Italian	Italiano	ee-ta-L-YA-no
Japanese	日本語	nee-HON-go
Korean	언어	u-nu
Mandarin	国语 (國語)	gwa ü
Polish	Polski	POL-skee
Portuguese	Português	por-too-GEYSH
Russian	Русский язык	ROOS-kee ya-ZIK
Spanish	Español	es-pan-YOL
Tagalog	Filipino	pee-lee-PEE-no
Thai	ภาษาไทย	PA-sa-tay
Ukrainian	Українська мова	oo-kra-YEEN-ska MO-va
Vietnamese	Tiếng Việt	dee-UNG VEE-ut

TABLE 3: WHAT COUNTRY ARE YOU FROM?

LANGUAGE	TRANSLATION	ENGLISH PRONUNCIATION
Arabic	من أي بلد انت؟	min ey be-led in-ta
Farsi	ديتسه یروشک هچ لها؟	æh-LE che kesh-VÆ-ree hæs-TEED?
French	De quel pays venez-vous?	du kel pe-YEE vu-ne-VOO
German	Von welchem Land kommen Sie?	fon VEL-KH-em lant KO-men zee?
Hindi	आप किस देश से हैं	op kis de-sha se HAY
Italian	Di dove è Lei (il paese)?	dee DO-ve E ley (eel pay-E-ze)?
Japanese	何処の国の人ですか？	do-ko no koo-nee no hee-to-des-ka
Korean	어느나라에서 왔나요?	u-noo-na-ra e-su WAT-su-yo?
Mandarin	您从哪国来(哪國來)的?	neen tsong na gwa lay du?
Polish	Od jaki kraj jest Pan (masc) Pani (fem)?	od ya-KEE kray YEST pan (masc) PA-nee (fem)
Portuguese	De que país é você?	jee KE PA-ees e vo-SE?
Russian	С какой старны вы?	s ka-KOY stra-NI vi?
Spanish	¿De donde es?	de DON-de es?
Tagalog	saang bansa ka galing	sa-ANG ban-SA ka GA-leeng
Thai	มาจากประเทศไหน?	mah juk pa-tayt nai?
Ukrainian	Ви з котрої країни?	vi z ko-TRO-yee kra-YEE-ni?
Vietnamese	Bạn đến từ nước nào ?	ban den tu nu-oc nau ?

TABLE 4: HELLO!

LANGUAGE	TRANSLATION	ENGLISH PRONUNCIATION
Arabic	مرحبا	MARR-ha-ba
Farsi	ملاس	sæ-LAM
French	Bonjour	bo*ng* ZHOO-kh
German	Hallo	HA-lo
Hindi	नमस्ते	na-ma-STE
Italian	Ciao	CHA-o
Japanese	こんにちは	kon-NEE-chee-wa
Korean	안녕하세요	an-NYUNG ha-se-yo
Mandarin	您好	neen hau
Polish	Dźień dobry	JEN DO-bree
Portuguese	Oi	OY
Russian	здравствуйте	z-DRAST-vooy-t-ye
Spanish	Hola	O-la
Tagalog	kamusta	ka-moos-TA
Thai	สวัสดี ครับ/ค่ะ	SA-wa-dee kap/ka
Ukrainian	Добрий день	DOB-ree den
Vietnamese	Xin chào	sin JAU

TABLE 5: PAIN?

LANGUAGE	TRANSLATION	ENGLISH PRONUNCIATION
Arabic	ألم	e-lam (wa-zha)
Farsi	درد	dærd
French	Douleur	doo-LUKH
German	Schmerz	sh-MER-ts
Hindi	दर्द	da-ER-da
Italian	Dolore	do-LO-re
Japanese	痛み	ee-ta-mee
Korean	고통 / 아픔	go-tong/a-poom
Mandarin	痛	tong
Polish	Ból	bool
Portuguese	Dor	dor
Russian	Боль	bol
Spanish	Dolor	do-LOR
Tagalog	Masakit	ma-sa-KEET
Thai	เจ็บ	jehp
Ukrainian	Біль	beel
Vietnamese	Đau	dau

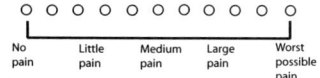

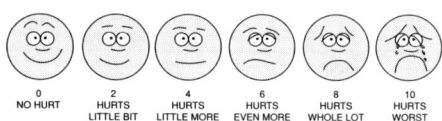

From Hockenberry MJ, Wilson D: *Wong's essentials of pediatric nursing*, ed. 8, St. Louis, 2009, Mosby. Used with permission. Copyright Mosby.

Arabic – عربي

WORD/PHRASE	TRANSLATION	ENGLISH PRONUNCIATION
Arabic	عربي	a-ra-BEE-ya
INTRODUCTION & REGISTRATION		
Hello	مرحبا	MARR-ha-ba
I am a doctor / nurse	أنا طبيبة/ممرضة	ana ta-BEEB (M-doctor) ta-BEE-ba (F-doctor) / ana moo-MARR-id (M-nurse), moo-MARR-ida (F-nurse)
What is your name?	ما اسمك؟	ma HOO-wa is-moo-ka?
Who is your doctor?	من هو طبيبك؟	men HOO-wa ta-BEEB bo-ka?
How old are you?	كم عمرك ؟	kam ÆM-ro-ka?
Birthdate?	تاريخ الميلاد؟	ta-REE-khe el- MEE-La-ad?
Telephone number?	رقم الهاتف؟	ra-kum el-ha-tif?
Address?	العنوان؟	el-ÆN-wan?
Social security number?	رقم الضمان الاجتماعي؟	ra-kum el-da-MAN el izh-te-MÆ-ee?
Insurance?	التأمين؟	el-TA-meen?
BASICS		
Do you understand?	هل تفهمني؟	hel fa-him-t?
Yes	نعم	NÆM
No	لا	La
Please	من فضلك	men-fud-luk
Thank you	شكرا	sho-kran

(cont.)

Sorry	آسف	Æ-sif
I don't understand	لا أفهم	la af-hem
Repeat	كرر	ka-rer
Speak slowly	تكلم ببطء	te-ka-lam bee-bu-tuh
Answer "yes" or "no"	أجب بـ "نعم" أو "لا"	ajeb bi NÆM au la
Here	هنا	hoon-a
This	هذا	had-da
It's alright (consoling)	كل شيء على ما يرام	kol-shey ala ma you-ram
I'll be right back	سأعود في الحال	sa-A au-ood fi el hal

GENERAL

What's wrong?	ما المشكلة ؟	ma el-mosh-kee-la?
Pain	ألم	a-lem
Do you have pain?	هل تشعر بالألم؟	hel tashour be a-lem?
Does the pain radiate?	هل الألم ينتشر ؟	hel el e-lam yant-ash-r?
Where (show me)	أين(أرني)	eyn-a (e-ree-nee)
Gone now	هل ال الم موجود الآن	hal el al-am ma-o-jood el an
Still present	مازال موجودا	ma za-la mau-zhoo-den
Sudden/gradual onset	بداية مفاجئة/ تدريجية	be-day-a moo-fa-je-a/ta-dree-jee-a
What bothers you the most?	بما تشكو؟	mem-ma tesh-koo?
Why did you come today?	لماذا جئت اليوم؟	lee-ma-za zhe-it il-ya-aum?

QUALITY		
If '0' is no pain and 10 is maximum pain, what number do you have now?	إذا كان '0' هو وعدم الشعور بالألم و10 هو أقصى قدر للشعور بالألم. حدد أحد الأرقام ؟	ee-za kan si-fer hoo-a ad-am el shoor be al-am we Æ-sh-ra ho-wa ak-sa ka-der men el a-lam, had-ed a-had el ar-kam ?
Burning	احتراق	E tee-rak
Constant	متوهج	moo-ta-waj
Dull	باهت	ba-hit
Intermittent	منقطع	moo-ta-ka-TÆ
Pressure	ضغط	DA-khit
Severe	حاد	had
Sharp/prickly	حاد /شائك	had/SHA-ik
Throbbing	خفقان	KHA-fa-kan
ASSOCIATED SYMPTOMS		
Onset during…(before/after)	بداية خلال… (قبل / بعد)	be-da-ya khe-lal (ka-bel / bÆ-de)…
Worse (with…)	أسوأ (مع …)	es-WA (ma…)
Better (with…)	أفضل (مع…)	UF-dul (ma…)
Cough	السعال	el su-ÆL
Deep breath	نفسا عميقا	nef-es-en a-mee-kan
Emotional upset	مشكلةعاطفية	mush-kee-la Æ-TE-fe-ya
Food	الطعام	el ta-ÆM
Movement	الحركة	el HA-ra-ka

(cont.)

Nothing	لا شيء	LA shey-an
Positioning	الوضع	el wad-Æ
Rest	الراحة	el ra-ha
Walking	المشي	el mesh-EE
TIME COURSE		
For how long?	إلى متى؟	EE-la mat-ta?
Today	اليوم	el yaum
Yesterday	أمس	EM-s
How many...	كم عدد...	kem a-dad ...
Months/weeks/days/hours/seconds	اشهر / اسابيع / أيام / ساعات / ثواني	esh-hor/es-a-bee-Æ/ey-yam/sa-ÆT/sa-WA-nee
Still present?	لا تزال موجودة؟	la ta-zal mau-zhoo-da
Gone now?	هل تشعر به الآن؟	hal ta-shoor be-hee el-an
How long did it last? (see Numbers)	كم من الوقت استمر الألم؟ (انظر الأرقام)	kem min el wakt est-mar al al-am
Have you had this before?	هل شعرت بهذا من قبل؟	hel sha-art be ha-da min-kab-l
How many times?	كم مرة؟	KEM ma-rra
When was the last time?	متى كانت آخر مرة؟	me-ta ka-net a-kher ma-ra
New	جديد	zhe-DEED
Old	قديم	KA-deem
CONTEXT		
Did you...?	هل...؟	hel...?
fall	وقعت	wa-kat?
trip	تعثرت	ta-tart?

faint	أغمي عليك	ukhe-mÆ e a-leyk?
twist	التويت	el-ta-weyt?
get hit	ضربت؟	doo-rebt?
get burned	تعرضت للحرق؟	ta-ar-adt la ha-rak?
get assaulted	تم الاعتداء عليك	tam el ee-teda-a a-leek?
get bitten	لدغت	loo-deg-t?

PAST MEDICAL HISTORY

Take medication?	هل تتناول الدواء؟	hel ta-ta-na-ool el de-wa?
(aspirin/antibiotics)	الأسبرين / المضادات الحيوية	(as-per-een/el moo-da-dat el ha-ya-WEE-ya)
Do you have (see Medical Problems)	هل لديك (انظر المشاكل الطبية)	hel le-DAY-ka…
allergies	الحساسية	el HAS-sa-see-ya
medical problems	مشاكل طبية	m-sha-kil too-bee-ya
…problems of the (see Body Parts)	… مشاكل (انظر أجزاء الجسم)	… m-sha-kil…

SURGICAL HISTORY

Have you had surgery?	هل تعرضت لعملية جراحية	hel ta-a-radt lee Æ-ma-lee-ya zhee-ra-HEE-ye
Surgery on…(see Body Parts)	جراحة في… (انظر أجزاء الجسم)	ZHEE-ra-ha fil…

SOCIAL HISTORY

Smoke?	هل تدخن؟	hel too-de-khen?
Drink?	هل تشرب؟	hel tesh-rab?
Take drugs?	هل تأخذ أدويه؟	hel te-e-khoz ed-wee-ya?

(cont.)

Recent travel?	هل سافرت مؤخرا؟	hel sa-fer-ta mo-a-kha-ran?
Are you sexually active?	هل أنت نشيط جنسيا؟	hel en-ta na-sheet zhin-see-yan?
Do you use condoms?	هل تستخدم الواقي الذكري؟	hel en-ta tes-ta-kha-dim el wa-kee el da-ka ree?
Homosexual	مثلي الجنس	mus-lee el-zhin-s

SYSTEMS REVIEW

Do you have...	هل لديكم...	hel le-dey-kom...

GENERAL

Fever	الحمى	el HUM-ma
Chills	ارجاف	ber-dee-ya
Weight loss	فقدان الوزن	fuk-dan el-wa-zen
Fatigue	تعب	TÆB
Sick contact	اتصال مع مرضى	it-tee-sal mÆ marr-da

HEENT

Sore throat	التهاب الحلق	il-tee-hab el HA-lik
Runny nose	سيلان الأنف	sa-ya-lan el en-if
Nosebleed	نزيف انفي	ne-zeef en-fee
Ear pain	ألم في الأذن	a-lem fee el-u-dun
Ear ringing	رنين في الأذن	re-neen fee el-u-dun
Decreased hearing	انخفاض في مستوى السمع	in-khee FAD fee must-a-wa el-sa-MÆ

EYE

Eye pain	الم في العين	a-lem fe el Æn
Blurry vision	عدم وضوح الرؤية	a-dam w-do- al roo-e-ya

Diplopia	رؤية مزدوجة	ruk-ya muz-da-wee-zha
Foreign body sensation	الشعور بجسم غريب في العين	eh-sas bee ha-zha KHA-reeba
Contact lenses	العدسات اللاصقه	el ÆH-de-set el la-SEE-ka
CARDIAC		
Chest pain	ألم في الصدر	a-lem fee el sad-r
Palpitations	خفقان	khe-fa-kat
Orthopnea	ضيق تنفس عند الاستلقاء	DEEK te-ne-fus Æ-yn-da el IS-til-KA-u
Dyspnea on exertion	ضيق تنفّس على الجهد المبذول	DEEK te-ne-fus a-la el zhe-hit el meb-dool
Fainting (syncope)	إغماء	el IKH-MÆ
Leg swelling	تورم في الرجل	ta-wa-room fee el ray-zhel
How many pillows?	كم وسادة؟	kem wee-sa-da?
PULMONARY		
Trouble breathing	متاعب في التنفس	me-ta-ÆB fee el te-ne-fus
SOB	ضيق تنفس	day-yuk el te-ne-fus
Cough	سعال	soo-ÆL
Sputum	لعاب	lo-ÆB
Pain on inspiration	ألم مع الشهيق	a-lem mÆ el-sha-heek
Hemoptysis	دم في اللعاب	dem fee el lo-ÆB
GI		
Abdominal pain	ألم في البطن	a-lem fee el-ba-TEN
Nausea	غثيان	KHA-sa-yan

(cont.)

Vomiting	قيء	kay
Vomiting blood	دم في القيء	dem fi el kay
Coffee ground emesis	بن في القيء	ben fi el kay
Anorexia	فقدان الشهية	fik-dan el sha-hee-ya
Diarrhea	إسهال	is-hal
Difficulty swallowing	صعوبة في البلع	SO-oo-ba fil be-LÆ
BRBPR	دم في الخروج	dem fee el khoo-roosh
Melena	خروج أسود	khoo-roosh ES-wed
Pain after eating	ألم بعد الأكل	a-lem BÆ-da el e-kel
Worms	ديدان	dee-dan
Constipation	إمساك	im-sak
GU		
Painful urination	تبول مؤلم	ta-ba-wol mu-lem
Urgent urination	تبول عاجل	ta-ba-wol Æ-zhel
Frequent urination	كثرة تبول	kis-rat ta-ba-wol
Bloody urination	تبول دموي	ta-ba-wol da-ma-wee
Discharge: vaginal/penile	التصريف: المهبلي / القضيبي	el TAS-reef : el MEH-be-lee/ el KA-dee-bee
PSYCH		
Anxiety	قلق	ka-lak
Depression	اكتئاب	EK-tee-ab
Suicidal thoughts	أفكار انتحارية	ef-kar in-tee-ha-ree-ya
Homicidal thoughts	أفكار تعدي على الغير	ef-kar TÆD-dee a-la el KHA-eer

Medication overdose	جرعه طبیة زائدة	jurah tebiah za-EE-da
Hear voices	هل تسمع أصواتا	hel tes-MÆ AS-wa-tan
NEURO		
Headache	صداع	SOO-DÆ
Worst headache of life	أسوأ صداع في الحياة	es-WÆ SOO-DÆ fil hay-yat
Weakness	ضعف	DÆF
Dizzy	مصاب بدوار	moo-SaB bee-da-war
What is your name?	ما هو اسمك؟	ma HOO-wa is-moo-ka?
Where are we?	أين نحن؟	ay-na NAH-noo?
What is the year/ month/date?	ما هي السنة / الشهر / التاريخ؟	ma hee-ya el se-na/el sha-her/el ta-reekh?
Bowel dysfunction	خلل في الأمعاء	kha-lel fee el em-Æ
Bladder dysfunction	اختلال وظیفي في المثانة	ikh-tee-lal wa-zee-fee fee el ma-sa-na
Photophobia	انزعاج من الضوء	in-zee-ÆZH min el DUK
Tingling/numbness	توخز / تخدر	ta-wa-khuz / ta-kha-dur
Decreased strength in...(See Body Part List)	انخفضت القوة في... (انظر لائحة أجزاء الجسم)	in-kha-fa-dat el koo-wa fee...
Seizure	صرع	sa-RÆ
Difficulty walking	صعوبة في المشي	SO-oo-ba fi el mash-ee
Difficulty speaking	صعوبة في النطق	SO-oo-ba fi el na-TIK
Spinning (vertigo)	دوار	doo-war
Confusion	تشويش	tash-weesh

(cont.)

MISC		
Lump	ورم	koot-la
Itching	حكاك	HOO-kak
Bruising	كدمه	kad-ma
Rash	طفح	TOF-ha
Swelling	ورم	wa-ram
Jaundice	يرقان	ya-ra-kan
GYNECOLOGIC		
Vaginal bleeding	نزيف مهبلي	na-zeef MA-ba-lee
Heavy	كثيف	ka-SEEF
Irregular	غير نظامي	khayr nee-za-mee-ya
Absent	غير موجود	g-heyr ma-o-JOOD
Vaginal discharge	تصريف مهبلي	tas-reef ma-ba-lee
Pelvic pain	ألم في الحوض	a-lem fil el HAWD
Rape	اغتصاب	ikh tee-SAB
Pain with intercourse	ألم عند الاتصال الجنسي	a-lem MÆ el i-tee-SAL el zhin-see
Contraceptive	وسائل منع الحمل	wa-sa-el me-NÆ el ha-MEL
OBSTETRIC		
Are you pregnant?	هل أنت حامل؟	hel in-tee ha-mel?
LMP how many days ago?	متى كانت أخر عادة شهرية لك	me-ta ka-net a-kher Æ-da sha-ree-ya le-kee?
Times pregnant?	كم مرة حملت؟	kem ma-ra HA-mel-tee?
Times delivered?	كم مرة ولدت؟	kem ma-ra wa-led-tee?
Miscarriage	إجهاض	izh-HAD

Abortion	إجهاض	izh-HAD
Fluid leakage	تسرب السوائل	TE-se-rob el sa-wa-il
Contraction	انكماش	IN-kee-mash
Fetal movement	حركة الجنين	ha-ra-ket el zhe-neen

TRAUMA

How many hours ago did you eat last?	متى كانت أخر مرة تناولت طعاما؟	me-ta ka-net a-kher ma-ra tanawalt ta'aman?
Lost consciousness?	هل فقدت وعيك ؟	hel fa-KUD-ta WÆ-ya-ka?
Tetanus within 5 years?	هل أصبت بالكزز في غضون الخمس السنوات الماضية؟	hel au-seb-ta b-l el ka-zaz fee KHE-soon el khem-s el sa-na-wat el ma-dee-ya

PEDIATRIC

How old?	كم عمره ؟	kem am-roo-hoo?
Vaccines up to date?	أحدث تطعيمات ؟	AH-DES ta-tee-mat?
Urinating normally	هل يبول طبيعيا	hel yu-ba-wel TA-bee-Æ-yen
Taking liquids	هل يأخذ السوائل	hel ye-khooz el sa-wa-il
Increased crying	هل هناك زيادة في البكاء	hel hoo-na-ka zee-ya-dat boo-ka-u
Ingestion	هل ابتلع شيئا	hel ib-te-la shey-en
FB	هل وضع شيئا داخله	hel wa-DÆ shey-en dekh-he-le-hoo
Premature	سابق لأوانه	sa-bik lee ee-wa-NEH
Birth complications	مضاعفات الولادة	moo-DA-Æ-fat el wee-la-da

(cont.)

PHYSICAL EXAM/INSTRUCTION		
Sit down (please)	اجلس (الرجاء)	izh-lis (re-zha-en)
Lie down	استلقي	is-tal-ki
Come here	تعال هنا	TÆL hoo-na
Relax	استريح	is-ta-REEH
Don't move	لا تتحرك	la te-ta ha-rak
Open your mouth	افتح فمك	if-TAH fa-moo-ka
Say "ahh"	قول "آه"	kol "ah"
Swallow	ابلع	ib-LÆ
Breath deeply	خذ نفسا عميقا	khoz na-fas-en Æ-mee-kun
Hold your breath	امسك نفسك	em-sook na-fas-soo-ka
Cough	اسعل	is-ÆL
Push	ادفع	id-FÆ
Pull	اسحب	is-HAB
Follow my finger	اتبع أصبعي	it-BÆ IS-BÆ-ay
Close your eyes	اغمض عينيك	akh-MID Æ-nay-ka
Smile	ابتسم	ib-tes-em
Can you feel this?	هل تشعر بهذا	hel tesh-OOR bee-ha-za
Copy this (movement)	قلد هذا (الحركة)	ka-led ha-za
I am going to put a finger in your rectum	سأضع أصبعي في المستقيم الخاصة بك	sa-a-DÆ is-BÆ-ee fee el moos-ta-keem el kha-SA bee-ka
I am going to examine your vagina	سأفحص مهبلك	sa-af-has meh-balek

REASSESSMENT		
Do you feel better?	هل تشعر بتحسن؟	hel tesh-OOR be ta-ha-soon
Do you feel worse?	هل تشعر بسوء؟	hel tesh-OOR es-wa
PATIENT WORDS		
I hurt	أشعر بألم	ashour be alam
Help!	ساعدوني!	sa-Æ-ee-doo-nee
Bathroom	الحمام	el ha-mam
Food	الطعام	el ta-ÆM
Water	الماء	el ma-e
PROCEDURES & CONSENT		
You need...	انك بحاجة إلى...	in-nee-ka bee-HÆ-zha il-la...
Injection	حقن	HU-kun
Stiches	قطب	koo-tab
Cast	مدلى	med-la
Crutches	عكازات	Æ-ka-zat
Perform surgery on (See Body Parts)	أداء جراحة (انظر أجزء الجسم)	ee da-e zhee-ra-HA...
The risks are...	المخاطر هي...	el ma-kha-ter hee-ya...
Bleeding	نزيف	na-zeef
Infection	عدوى	ÆD-wa
Scar	ندبة	ned-ba
Repeat procedure	تكرار الإجراء	tik-rar el izh-ra
Iodine	اليود	el yood

(cont.)

Damage to (see Body Parts)	ضرر في	DA-rar fee
Sign here	وقع هنا	wa-KÆ hoo-na
TESTS		
X-ray	أشعه اكس X	e-sha-X
C.A.T. Scan	أشعه المقطعية	e-sha-Æ el mok-ta-Æ-ya
Ultrasound	الاشعه الفوق الصوتية	el e-sha-Æ el fawk el saw-tee-a
Catheterization/bladder catheter	القسطرة / القسطرة في المثانه	el ka-ster-a / el ka-ster-a fil ma-sA-na
Colonoscopy	ناظور	na-ZOOR
Endoscopy	تنظير داخليّ	tan-ZEER da-khee-lee
END OF LIFE		
Do you want us to...	هل تريد منا القيام بـ...	hel too-reed min-na...
Perform CPR	أداء الإسعافات الأولية	e-da el es-Æ-fat el au-oo-lee-ya
Defibrillate		دفيبريلّت
Intubate	أدخل أنبوب	ed-khol in-boob
He/she is dead	إنه ميت	In-a-hoo mey-yet
We did all we could	لقد فعلنا كل ما في وسعنا	la-kad fa-ÆL-na kol ma fee wi-SÆ-ee-na
DISCHARGE		
You have... (See Medical Prob List)	لديك...	le-dey-ka...
He/she is going to stay in the hospital	انه سيبقى في المستشفى	in-na-hoo sa-yeb-ka fil moos-stash-fa

Take "X" pills "Y" times a day for "Z" days	خذ مرات يومياً لمدة "Z" أيام "Y" حبوب "X"	khooz "X" ha-boob "Y" ma-rat ya-oo-mee-an i-moo-dat "Z" ay-yam
Pills	حبوب	hoo-boob
Antibiotics	المضادات الحيوية	el moo-da-dat el ha-ya-WEE-ya
Before/after meals	قبل / بعد الوجبات	ka-bil / BÆD el wazh-bat
Return to the ER if…	عد إلى الطوارئ إذا…	ÆD ee-la el TA-wa-ri-u iza…
Follow up at "X" on "Y"	متابعة في"X" على "Y"	moo-ta-BÆ fee "X", "Y".
You're welcome	مرحبا بك	mara-HEB-n bee-ka
Goodbye	وداعا	wa-DÆN
MEDICAL PROBS		
AIDS/HIV	الإيدز / فيروس نقص المناعة المكتسبة	el eyds / fee-roos nuks el ma-NÆ al muktasba
Anemia	فقر في الدم	fu-kor fil dem
Arrhythmia	دقات قلب غير منتظمة	da-KAT KA-lub KHA-eer mun-ta-zee-ma
Arthritis	روماتيزم	roo-ma-teez-ma
Asthma	ربو	re-bu
Bronchitis	التهاب رئوي	il-tee-hab ree-au-wee
Cancer	سرطان	sa-ra-tan
Cirrhosis	تليّف كبديّ	tel-ley-yoof kib-dee
Cholesterol	الكولسترول	el ko-les-ter-ol
Cold	برد	ba-red
Constipation	إمساك	im-sak

(cont.)

Cyst	مثانة	ma-sA-na
Diabetes	مرض السكر	ma-rad el sook-ar
Dialysis	غسل الكلية	KHA-sil el koo-lee-ya
Diverticulitis	التهاب في المصران	il-tee-hab fee el MUS-ran
Emphysema	انتفاخ رئة	in-tee-fakh ree-a
Fibroids	تليف	te-ley-uf
Fracture	كسر	kis-er
Flu	أنفلونزا	in-flu-en-za
Gallstones	حصاة صفراويّة	hoo-SAT SUF-ra-wee-ya
Gastritis/GERD	التهاب المعدة	il-tee-hab el MÆ-ee-da
Hepatitis	التهاب الكبد	il-tee-hab el ka-bid
Heart attack	حركة قلبية	ha-ra-ka kal-bee-ya
Heart disease	أمراض القلب	am-rad el kalb
Heart failure	فشل القلب	fa-shel el kalb
Hypertension	ارتفاع ضغط الدم	ir-tee-FÆ DAKHT el dam
Indigestion	عسر الهضم	a-ser el had-im
Kidney stone	حجارة في الكلية	HEE-zha-ram fil keel-ya
Lupus	الذئبه	el ze-ba
Migraine	داء الشقيقة	da-e el sha-kee-ka
Murmur	دندنة	den-den-a
Pacemaker	منظم القلب	moo-na-zem el ka-lib
Pneumonia	التهاب رئويّ	il-tee-hab ree-au-wee
Seizures	صرع	Sa-RÆ

STD	الأمراض التي تنتقل بالاتصال الجنسي	el am-rad el le-tee ten-tau-kel bil el i-tee-sal el zhin-see
Stroke	سكته	sek-ta
Ulcer	قرحة	kar-HÆ
Ulcerative colitis	التهاب القولون	il-tee-hab el ko-lon
UTI	التهاب في المسالك البولية	il-tee-hab fee el ma-sa-leek el bau-lee-ya
BODY PARTS		
Abdomen	البطن	el ba-tin
Ankle	الكاحل	el ka-HIL
Appendix	الزائدة الدودية	el za-ee-da el-doo-day-ya
Arm	الذراع	el zoo-RÆ
Artery	الشريان	el shoo-ree-yan
Back	الظهر	el ZA-her
Bladder	المثانة	el ma-sa-na
Blood	الدم	el dem
Bone	العظم	el ÆZM
Brain	المخ	el mookh
Breast	الثدي	el sa-dee
Calf	بطة القدم	bu-tu el KA-dem
Chest	الصدر	el SADR
Chin	الذقن	el da-kin
Ear	الأذن	el oo-dun

(cont.)

Elbow	الكوع	el koo-Æ
Eye	العين	el Æ-yen
Face	الوجه	el wazh-ha
Finger	الإصبع	el IS-BÆ
Foot	القدم	el ka-dom
Hand	اليد	el yed
Head	الرأس	el ra-e-s
Heart	القلب	el kulb
Gallbladder	المرارة	el ma-ra-ra
Jaw	الفك	el fak
Joint	المفصل	el maf-sal
Kidney	الكلية	el keel-ya
Knee	الركبة	el ruk-a-ba
Leg	الساق	el sak
Liver	الكبد	el ka-bid
Mouth	الفم	el fam
Muscle	العضل	el ÆDL
Neck	الرقبة	el rak-ba
Nerve	العصب	el Æ-SUB
Nose	الأنف	el Æ-nif
Ovary	المبيض	el ma-BEED
Pancreas	البنكرياس	el pan-kree-es
Penis	القضيب	el ka-DEEB

Prostate	البروستاتة	el pro-stat
Rectum	المستقيم	el mos-ta-keem
Rib	الضلع	el DO-LÆ
Shoulder	الكتف	el ke-tif
Skin	الجلد	el zhe-led
Spleen	الطحال	el TO-HAL
Spine	العمود الفقري	el Æ-mood el fu-ka-ree
Stomach	المعدة	el MÆ-da
Teeth	الأسنان	el es-nan
Testicle	الخصية	el khes-ya
Throat	الحنجرة	el HON-zha-ra
Thyroid	الغدة الدرقية	el KHOO-da el da-ra-kee-ya
Toe	إصبع القدم	is-BÆ el ka-dum
Tonsils	لوز الحلق	lauz el ha-luk
Tongue	اللسان	el lee-san
Uterus	الرحم	el ra-hem
Vagina	المهبل	el mah-bel
Vein	المنوال	el min-wal
Wrist	المعصم	el MÆ-sam

(cont.)

NUMBERS

How many (times)?	كم مرة ؟	kem ma-ra
0	صفر	SI-fer
1	واحد	wa-HID
2	اثنين	IS-neyn
3	ثلاثة	se-la-sa
4	أربعة	ar-BÆ
5	خمسة	khem-sa
6	ستة	sit-ta
7	سبعة	sa-BÆ
8	ثمانية	se-man-ee-ya
9	تسعة	ti-SÆ
10	عشر	ÆSH-ra
11	أحد عشر	IH-da Æ-sher
20	عشرون	ÆSH-roon
30	ثلائون	sa-la-soon
40	أربعون	er-ba-Æ-ee-n
50	خمسون	khem-soon
60	ستون	sit-oon
70	سبعون	SEB-oon
80	ثمانون	se-me-noon
90	تسعون	tis-OON
100	مائة	mee-a

Farsi (Persian) – فارسی

WORD/PHRASE	TRANSLATION	ENGLISH PRONUNCIATION
Farsi	فارسی	far-SEE
INTRODUCTION & REGISTRATION		
Hello	سلام	sæ-LAM
I am doctor/nurse (add your name)	من دکتر/پرستار ــــ هستم	mæn dok-TOR (doctor) / pæ-ræs-TAR (nurse) (add your name) hæs-TÆM
What is your name?	اسم شما چیه؟	ES-me sho-MA CHEE-ye?
Who is your doctor?	دکتر شما کیه؟	dok-TO-re sho-MA KEE-ye?
How old are you?	شما چند سالتونه؟	sho-MA chænd sa-le-TOO-ne?
Birthdate?	تاریخ تولد؟	ta-REE-khe tæ-VÆ-lod?
Telephone number?	شماره تلفن؟	sho-MA-re-ye te-le-FON?
Address?	آدرس؟	ad-RES?
Social security number?	شماره سوشیال سکوریتی؟	sho-MA-re-ye "social security"
Insurance?	بیمه؟	bee-ME?
BASICS		
Do you understand?	میفهمید؟	mee-FÆH-meed?
Yes	بله	BÆ-le
No	نه	næ
Please	لطفا	lot-FÆN
Thank you	ممنون	mæm-NOON
Sorry	ببخشید	BE-bækh-sheed

(cont.)

I don't understand	نمیفهمم	NE-mee-fæh-mæm
Repeat	تکرار کنید	tek-RAR ko-NEED
Speak slowly	آهسته صحبت کنید	a-HES-te soh-BÆT ko-NEED
Answer "yes" or "no"	بله یا نه	BÆ-le ya næ
Here	اینجا	een-JA
This	این	een
It's alright (consoling)	چیزی نیست	CHEE-zee neest
I'll be right back	الآن برمیگردم	æl-AN BÆR-mee-gær-dæm

GENERAL

What's wrong?	مشکل چیه؟	mosh-KEL CHEE-ye?
Pain	درد	dærd
Do you have pain?	درد دارید؟	dærd da-REED?
Does the pain radiate?	آیا این درد به جایی میزند؟	a-YA een dærd be JA-yee mee-zæ-næd?
Where (show me)	کجا (ببینم)	ko-JA? (BE-bee-næm)
Gone now	حالا رفت	HA-la ræft
Still present	هنوز هست	hæ-NOOZ hæst
Sudden/gradual onset	شروع ناگهانی/تدریجی	sho-ROO-e NA-gæ-ha-nee/tæd-ree-JEE
What bothers you the most?	چه چیزی بیشتر اذیتتان میکند؟	che CHEE-zee beesh-TÆR æz-YÆ-te-tan mee-ko-NÆD?
Why did you come today?	چرا امروز آمدید؟	CHE-ra em-ROOZ a-mæ-DEED?

Farsi (Persian) – فارسی

QUALITY		
If '0' is no pain and 10 is maximum pain, what number do you have now?	از صفر، با بدون درد تا ده یا حداکثر درد چه قدر درد دارید؟	æz sef-r ya be-DOO-ne dærd ta dæh ya hæ-DE æk-SÆR dærd, che gæd-r dærd da-REED?
Burning	سوزش	soo-ZESH
Constant	دائم	da-EM
Dull	مرده درد	mor-de-DÆRD
Intermittent	گهگاهی	gæh-ga-HEE
Pressure	فشار	fe-SHAR
Severe	شديد	shæ-DEED
Sharp/prickly	تيز	teez
Throbbing	با تپش	ba tæ-PESH
ASSOCIATED SYMPTOMS		
Onset during ___ (before/after)	شروع هنگام ___ (قبل/بعد)	sho-ROO hen-GA-me ___ (gæb-l/bæd)
Worse (with ___)	بدتر (با ___)	BÆD-tær (ba ___)
Better (with ___)	بهتر (با ___)	BEH-tær (ba ___)
Cough	سرفه	sor-FE
Deep breath	نفس عميق	næ-FÆ-se æ-MEEG
Emotional upset	ناراحتی احساسی	na-ra-hæ-TEE-ye eh-SA-see
Food	غذا	gæ-ZA
Movement	حركت	hæ-re-KÆT
Nothing	هيچى	HEE-chee

(cont.)

Positioning	طرز قرار گرفتن	TÆR-ze gæ-RAR ge-ref-TÆN
Rest	استراحت	ES-TE-RA-HÆT
Walking	راه رفتن	rah ræf-TÆN
TIME COURSE		
For how long?	برای چند وقت؟	bæ-RA-ye chænd væg-t?
Today	امروز	em-ROOZ
Yesterday	دیروز	dee-ROOZ
How many ___	چند تا ___	chænd ta ___?
Months/weeks/days/ hours/seconds	ماهها/هفتهها/روزها/ ساعتها/ ثانیهها	
Still present?	هنوز هست؟	hæ-NOOZ hæst?
Gone now?	حالا رفت؟	HA-la ræft?
How long did it last? (see Numbers)	چه قدر طول کشید؟	che gæd-r tool ke-SHEED?
Have you had this before?	قبلا هم این را داشتهاید؟	gæb-LÆN hæm een ra dash-TE-eed?
How many times?	چند دفعه؟	chænd dæf-E?
When was the last time?	دفعه قبل کی بود؟	DÆF-E-YE GÆB-L KEY BOOD?
New	تازه	ta-ZE
Old	کهنه	koh-NE
CONTEXT		
Did you ___?	آیا ___؟	a-YA ___?
fall	افتادید	of-TA-deed
trip	لیز خوردید	leez khor-DEED
faint	غش کردید	gæsh kær-DEED

twist	پیچ خورد	peech khord
get hit	ضربه خوردید	zær-BE khor-DEED
get burned	سوختید	SOOKH-TEED
get assaulted	به شما تجاوز شد	be sho-MA tæ-ja-VOZ shod
get bitten	گازتان گرفتند	ga-ze-TAN ge-ref-TÆN-D
PAST MEDICAL HISTORY		
Take medication?	دارو مصرف میکنید؟	da-roo mæs-RÆF mee-ko-NEED?
(aspirin/antibiotics)	(آسپیرین/آنتیبیوتیک)	(as-pee-REEN/AN-tee-BEE-yo-teek)
Do you have ___ (see Medical Problems)	آیا ___ دارید	a-YA ___ da-REED?
allergies	آلرژی	A-LER-ZHEE
medical problems	مشکلات پزشکی	mosh-ke-LA-te pe-zesh-KEE
___problems of the (see Body Parts)	مشکلات ___	___ mosh-ke-LA-te
SURGICAL HISTORY		
Have you had surgery?	تا به حال عمل جراحی داشته‌اید؟	ta be hal æ-MÆ-le jæ-ra-HEE dash-te-EED?
Surgery on ___ (see Body Parts)	عمل ___	æ-MA-le ___
Social History		
Smoke?	سیگار میکشید؟	see-GAR mee-ke-SHEED?
Drink?	مشروب می نوشید؟	mash-ROOB mee-noo-SHEED?
Take drugs?	مواد مخدر مصرف میکنید؟	mæ-VA-de mo-khæ-DER mæs-RÆF mee-ko-NEED?

(cont.)

Recent travel?	اخیراً سفر کردید؟	æ-khee-RÆN sæ-FÆR kær-DEED?
Are you sexually active?	آیا فعالیت جنسی دارید؟	A-YA FÆ-A-LEE-YA-TE JEN-SEE DA-REED?
Do you use condoms?	کاندوم استفاده میکنید؟	kan-DOM es-te-FA-de mee-ko-NEED?
Homosexual	همجنسگرا	HAM-JENS-GÆ-RA

SYSTEMS REVIEW

Do you have___	___ دارید	___ da-REED?

GENERAL

Fever	تب	tæb
Chills	لرز	lærz
Weight loss	کاهش وزن	KA-HE-SHE VÆZ-N
Fatigue	خستگی	khæs-te-GEE
Sick contact	تماس با بیمار	tæ-MAS ba bee-MAR

HEENT

Sore throat	گلودرد	gæ-loo-DÆRD
Runny nose	آبریزش بینی	ab-ree-ZE-she bee-NEE
Nosebleed	خونریزی بینی	khoon-ree-ZEE-ye bee-NEE
Ear pain	گوشدرد	GOOSH-DÆRD
Ear ringing	وزوز گوش	vez-VE-ze goosh
Decreased hearing	کاهش شنوایی	ka-he-SHE she-næ-va-YEE

EYE

Eye pain	چشم‌درد	chesh-m-DÆRD

Blurry vision	تاری دید	ta-REE-ye deed
Diplopia	دوبینی (دوتایی دیدن)	DO-BEE-NEE (do-ta-YEE dee-DÆN)
Foreign body sensation	احساس جسم خارجی	eh-SA-se JES-me kha-re-JEE
Contact lenses	لنز	lenz

CARDIAC

Chest pain	درد سینه	dær-DE see-NE
Palpitations	تپش قلب	tæ-pe-SHE gæl-b
Orthopnea	تنگی نفس هنگام ایستادن	tæn-GEE-ye næ-FÆS hen-GA-me ees-ta-DÆN
Dyspnea on exertion	تنگی نفس هنگام فعالیت	tæn-GEE-ye næ-FÆS hen-GA-me fæ-a-lee-YAT
Fainting (syncope)	غش (سنکوب)	GÆSH (sæn-KOB)
Leg swelling	ورم پا	væ-RÆ-me pa
How many pillows?	چند تا بالش؟	chænd ta ba-LESH?

PULMONARY

Trouble breathing	سختی تنفس	sækh-TEE-ye tæ-næ-FOS
SOB	تنگی نفس	tæn-GEE-ye næ-FÆS
Cough	سرفه	sor-FE
Sputum	خلط	KHEL-T
Pain on inspiration	درد هنگام دم	dærd hen-GA-me dæm
Hemoptysis	خونریزی هنگام سرفه	khoon-ree-ZEE hen-GA-me sor-FE

GI

Abdominal pain	درد شکم	dær-DE she-KÆM

Farsi (Persian) – فارسی

Nausea	تهوع	tæ-hæ-VO
Vomiting	استفراغ	es-tef-RAG
Vomiting blood	استفراغ خونی	es-tef-RA-ge khoo-NEE
Coffee ground emesis	استفراغ قهوهای رنگ	es-tef-RA-ge gæh-ve-EE ræng
Anorexia	بیاشتهایی	bee-esh-te-ha-YEE
Diarrhea	اسهال	es-HAL
Difficulty swallowing	سختی در قورت دادن	sækh-TEE dær goor-t da-DÆN
BRBPR	خونریزی روشن از مقعد	khoon-ree-ZEE-ye ro-SHÆN æz mæg-ÆD
Melena	خونریزی سیاه از مقعد	khoon-reeZEE-ye see-YAH æz mæg-ÆD
Pain after eating	درد بعد از غذا	DÆRD BÆD ÆZ GÆ-ZA
Worms	کرم	kerm
Constipation	یبوست	yo-boo-SÆT
GU		
Painful urination	درد ادرار	dær-DE ed-RAR
Urgent urination	ادرار اضطراری	ed-RA-re ez-te-ra-REE
Frequent urination	تکرر ادرار	TÆ-KÆ-RO-RE ED-RAR
Bloody urination	ادرار خونی	ed-RA-re khoo-NEE
Discharge: vaginal/penile	ترشح واژن/آلت	tæ-ræ-SHO-he va-ZHÆN/a-LÆT
PSYCH		
Anxiety	اضطراب	ez-te-RAB
Depression	افسردگی	æf-sor-de-GEE

Farsi (Persian) – فارسی

Suicidal thoughts	افکار خودکشی	æf-KA-re khod-ko-SHEE
Homicidal thoughts	افکار قتل	ÆF-KA-RE GÆT-L
Medication overdose	مصرف بیش از حد دارو	mæs-RÆ-fe beesh æz HÆ-de da-ROO
Hear voices	صداهای غیرعادی	se-da-HA-ye GEY-re a-DEE
NEURO		
Headache	سردرد	sær-DÆRD
Worst headache of life	بدترین سردرد ممکن	bæd-tæ-REEN sær-DÆR-de mom-KEN
Weakness	ضعف	zæf
Dizzy	گیج	geej
What is your name?	اسم شما چیه؟	ES-me sho-MA CHEE-ye?
Where are we?	ما کجاییم؟	ma ko-JA-yeem?
What is the year/month/date?	الآن چه سالیه/ماهیه/روزیه؟	æl-AN che SA-lee-ye/MA-hee-ye/ROO-zee-ye?
Bowel dysfunction	اختلال گوارشی	ekh-te-LA-le go-va-re-SHEE
Bladder dysfunction	اختلال مثانه	ekh-te-LA-le mæ-sa-NE
Photophobia	ترس از نور	tærs æz noor
Tingling/numbness	گزگز/بیحسی	gez gez/bee-he-SEE
Decreased strength in…(See Body Part List)	احساس ضعف در ___	eh-SA-se zæf dær ___
Seizure	تشنج	tæ-shæ-NOJ
Difficulty walking	مشکل راه رفتن	mosh-KE-le rah ræf-TÆN
Difficulty speaking	مشکل حرف زدن	mosh-KE-le hærf zæ-DÆN

Spinning (vertigo)	سرگیجه	saer-gee-JE
Confusion	گیجی	gee-JEE
MISC		
Lump	توده	too-DE
Itching	خارش	kha-RESH
Bruising	کبودی	kæ-boo-DEE
Rash	دانه زدن	da-NE zæ-DÆN
Swelling	تورم	tæ-væ-ROM
Jaundice	زردی	zær-DEE
GYNECOLOGIC		
Vaginal bleeding	خونریزی واژن	khoon-ree-ZEE-ye va-ZHÆN
Heavy	سنگین	sæn-GEEN
Irregular	نامنظم	na-mo-næ-ZÆM
Absent	نداشتن	næ-dash-TÆN
Vaginal discharge	ترشح واژن	tæ-ræ-SHO-he va-ZHÆN
Pelvic pain	درد لگن	dær-DE læ-GÆN
Rape	تجاوز جنسی	tæ-ja-VO-ze jen-SEE
Pain with intercourse	درد هنگام نزدیکی	dærd hen-GA-me næz-dee-KEE
Contraceptive	ضد بارداری	ze-DE bar-da-REE
OBSTETRIC		
Are you pregnant?	حامله هستید؟	ha-me-LE hæs-TEED?
LMP how many days ago?	آخرین بار کی پریود شدید؟	a-khæ-REEN bar key pe-ree-YOD sho-DEED?

Farsi (Persian) – فارسی

Times pregnant?	چند بار حامله بودید؟	chænd bar ha-me-LE boo-DEED?
Times delivered?	چند بار زایمان کردید؟	chænd bar zay-MAN kær-DEED?
Miscarriage	سقط	seg-t
Abortion	سقط	seg-t
Fluid leakage	ترشح آبکی	tæ-ræ-SHO-he a-bæ-KEE
Contraction	انقباض	en-ge-BAZ
Fetal movement	حرکت جنین	hæ-re-KÆ-te jæ-NEEN
TRAUMA		
How many hours ago did you eat last?	آخرین بار کی غذا خوردید؟	a-khæ-REEN bar key gæ-ZA khor-DEED?
Lost consciousness?	هوشیاری خود را از دست	hoosh-ya-REE-ye khod ra æz dæst da-DEED?
Tetanus within 5 years?	کزاز در پنج سال اخیر؟	ko-ZAZ dær pæn-j SA-le æ-KHEER?
PEDIATRIC		
How old?	چند سال؟	chænd sal?
Vaccines up to date?	همه واکسنها را زدید؟	hæ-ME-ye vak-SÆN-ha ra zæ-DEED?
Urinating normally	ادرار معمولی	ed-RA-re mæ-moo-LEE
Taking liquids	نوشیدن مایعات	noo-shee-DÆ-ne ma-ye-AT
Increased crying	زیاد گریه کردن	zee-YAD ger-YE kær-DÆN
Ingestion	وارد شدن غذا	va-RED sho-DÆ-ne gæ-ZA
Foreign body	جسم خارجی	jes-ME kha-re-JEE

(cont.)

Farsi (Persian) – فارسی

Premature	زودرس	zood-RÆS
Birth complications	عوارض زایمان	æ-va-RE-ze zay-MAN
PHYSICAL EXAM/INSTRUCTION		
Sit down (please)	(لطفاً) بنشینید	(lot-FÆN) ben-shee-NEED
Lie down	دراز بکشید	de-RAZ be-ke-SHEED
Come here	اینجا بیایید	een-JA bee-ya-YEED
Relax	خودتان را شل کنید	kho-de-TAN ra shol ko-NEED
Don't move	تکان نخورید	te-KAN næ-kho-REED
Open your mouth	دهانتان را باز کنید	dæ-HA-ne-tan ra baz ko-NEED
Say "ahh"	بگو "آ"	be-GOO "ahh"
Swallow	قورت بدهید	goor-t be-dæ-HEED
Breath deeply	نفس عمیق	næ-FÆ-se æ-MEEG
Hold your breath	نفستان را نگه دارید	næ-FÆ-se-tan ra ne-GÆH da-REED
Cough	سرفه	sor-FE
Push	هل بدهید	hol be-dæ-HEED
Pull	بکشید	be-ke-SHEED
Follow my finger	انگشت من را دنبال کنید	æn-GOSH-te mæn ra don-BAL ko-NEED
Close your eyes	چشمانتان را ببندید	chesh-MA-ne-tan ra be-bæn-DEED
Smile	لبخند	læb-KHÆND
Can you feel this?	حس میکنید؟	hes mee-ko-NEED?
Copy this (movement)	همین کار را بکنید	hæ-MEEN kar ra be-ko-NEED

English	فارسی	Pronunciation
I am going to put a finger in your rectum	می خواهم از مقعد شما را معاینه	mee-kha-HÆM æz mæ-GÆD sho-MA ra mo-a-ye-NE ko-NÆM
I am going to examine your vagina	میخواهم از جلو شما را معاینه	

REASSESSMENT

Do you feel better?	بهتر شدید؟	beh-TÆR sho-DEED?
Do you feel worse?	بدتر شدید؟	bæd-TÆR sho-DEED?

PATIENT WORDS

I hurt	درد دارم	dærd da-RÆM
Help!	کمک	ko-MÆK!
Bathroom	دستشویی	dæst-shoo-YEE
Food	غذا	gæ-ZA
Water	آب	ab

PROCEDURES & CONSENT

You need...	شما ... احتیاج دارید	sho-MA ... eh-tee-YAJ da-REED
Injection	تزریق	tæz-REEG
Stitches	بخیه	bæ-khee-YE
Cast	گچ	gæch
Crutches	عصا	æ-SA
Perform surgery on (See Body Parts)___	عمل جراحی ___	æ-mæ-LE jæ-ra-HEE ___
The risks are___	خطرها ___ است	khæ-tær-HA ___ æst
Bleeding	خونریزی	khoon-ree-ZEE

(cont.)

Infection	عفونت	o-foo-NÆT
Scar	جای جوش خوردن زخم	ja-YE joosh khor-DÆ-ne zækh-m
Repeat procedure	تکرار عمل	tek-RA-re æ-MÆL
Iodine	ید	yod
Damage to___ (see Body Parts)	صدمه به___	sæ-dæ-ME be ___
Sign here	اینجا را امضا کنید	een-JA ra em-ZA ko-NEED

TESTS

X-ray	ایکس ری	eeks rey
C.A.T. Scan	سی تی اسکن	see tee es-KÆN
Ultrasound	سونوگرافی	so-nog-RA-fee
Catheterization/ bladder catheter	سوند زدن/سوند مثانه	sond zæ-DÆN/son-DE mæ-sa-NE
Colonoscopy	کلنوسکپی	co-lo-NOS-ko-pee
Endoscopy	آندوسکپی	an-DOS-ko-pee

END OF LIFE

Do you want us to___	آیا میخواهید که ما___	a-YA mee-kha-HEED ke ma ___
Perform CPR	ماساژ قلبی بدهیم	ma-sa-ZHE gæl-BEE be-dæ-HEEM
Defibrillate	شما را به دستگاه وصل کنیم	sho-MA ra be dæst-GAH væs-l ko-NEEM?
Intubate	لوله بگذاریم	loo-LE be-go-za-REEM
He/she is dead	تمام کردند	tæ-MAM kær-DÆND
We did all we could	ما هر کاری میتونستیم کردیم	ma hær KA-ree mee-too-nes-TEEM kær-DEEM

Farsi (Persian) – فارسی

DISCHARGE		
You have___ (See Medical Prob List)	شما ___ دارید	sho-MA ... da-REED
He/she is going to stay in the hospital	میخواهد در بیمارستان بماند	mee-kha-HÆD dær bee-ma-res-TAN be-ma-NÆD
Take "X" pills "Y" times a day for "Z" days	عدد برای "Y" قرص "X" روزی "Z"	"X" gors, roo-ZEE "Y" æ-DÆD, bæ-RA-ye "Z" rooz
Pills	قرص	gor-s
Antibiotics	آنتی بیوتیک	AN-tee-BEE-yo-teek
Before/after meals	قبل/بعدازغذا	gæb-l/bæd æz gæ-ZA
Return to the ER if___	به اورژانس برگردید اگر ___	be oor-ZHANS bær-gær-DEED æ-GÆR___
Follow up at "X" on "Y"	مراجعه کنید "Y" به "X" روز	roo-ZE "X" be "Y" mo-ra-je-E ko-NEED
You're welcome	خواهش میکنم	kha-HESH mee-ko-NÆM
Goodbye	خداحافظ	kho-da-HA-fez

MEDICAL PROBS		
AIDS/HIV	ایدز	eydz
Anemia	کمخونی	kæm-khoo-NEE
Arrhythmia	ریتم بد قلب	REET-me BÆ-de gæl-b
Arthritis	آرترز	ar-to-ROZ
Asthma	آسم	as-m
Bronchitis	برونشیت	bron-SHEET
Cancer	سرطان	sæ-ræ-TAN
Cirrhosis	سیروز	see-ROZ
Cholesterol	کلسترل	ko-les-te-ROL

Farsi (Persian) – فارسی

Cold	سرماخوردگی	sær-ma-khor-DE-gee
Constipation	یبوست	yo-boo-SÆT
Cyst	کیست	keest
Diabetes	دیابت	dee-ya-BET
Dialysis	دیالیز	dee-ya-LEEZ
Diverticulitis	دیورتیکولیت	dee-ver-tee-koo-LEET
Emphysema	آمفیزم	am-fee-ZEM
Fibroids	فیبروم	feeb-ROM
Fracture	شکستگی	she-kæs-te-GEE
Flu	آنفلانزا	an-fe-lan-ZA
Gallstones	سنگ کیسه صفرا	sæn-GE kee-SE sæf-RA
Gastritis/GERD	ورم معده/برگرداندن غذا	væ-ræ-ME me-DE/bær-gær-dan-DÆ-ne gæ-ZA
Hepatitis	هپاتیت	he-pa-TEET
Heart attack	حمله قلبی	hæm-LE-ye gæl-BEE
Heart disease	ناراحتی قلبی	na-ra-hæ-TEE-ye gæl-BEE
Heart failure	نارسایی قلبی	na-ræ-sa-YEE-ye gæl-BEE
Hypertension	فشار خون بالا	fe-SHA-re KHOO-ne ba-LA
Indigestion	سوء هضم	soo-E hæzm
Kidney stone	سنگ کلیه	san-GE ko-lee-YE
Lupus	لوپوس	loo-POOS
Migraine	میگرن	meeg-REN
Murmur	سوفل	SOOF-lu

Farsi (Persian) – فارسی

Pacemaker	پیسمیکر/دستگاه محرک قلب	peys-mey-KER/dæst-GA-he mo-hæ-RE-ke gælb
Pneumonia	ذات‌الریه	za-tol-ree-YE
Seizures	تشنج	tæ-shæ-NOJ
STD	بیماری مقاربی	bee-ma-REE-ye mo-gæ-re-BEE
Stroke	سکته مغزی	sek-TE-ye mæg-ZEE
Ulcer	زخم	zækh-m
Ulcerative colitis	کولیت اولسروز	ko-LEE-te ool-se-ROZ
UTI	عفونت ادراری	o-foo-NÆ-te ed-ra-REE
BODY PARTS		
Abdomen	شکم	she-KÆM
Ankle	قوزک	goo-ZÆK
Appendix	آپاندیس	a-pan-DEES
Arm	بازو	ba-ZOO
Artery	شریان/سرخرگ	shæ-ree-YAN/sor-kh-RÆG
Back	کمر	kæ-MÆR
Bladder	مثانه	mæ-sa-NE
Blood	خون	khoon
Bone	استخوان	os-to-KHAN
Brain	مغز	mæg-z
Breast	پستان	pes-TAN
Calf	ساق پا	SA-ge pa
Chest	سینه	see-NE

(cont.)

Chin	چانه	cha-NE
Ear	گوش	goosh
Elbow	آرنج	a-REN-J
Eye	چشم	chesh-m
Face	صورت	soo-RÆT
Finger	انگشت	æn-GOSH-T
Foot	پا (پایین پا)	pa (pa-YEE-ne pa)
Hand	دست	dæst
Head	سر	sær
Heart	قلب	gæl-b
Gallbladder	کیسه صفرا	kee-SE sæf-RA
Jaw	فک	fæk
Joint	مفصل	mæf-SÆL
Kidney	کلیه	ko-lee-YE
Knee	زانو	za-NOO
Leg	پا	pa
Liver	کبد	kæ-BED
Mouth	دهان	dæ-HAN
Muscle	ماهیچه	ma-hee-CHE
Neck	گردن	gær-DÆN
Nerve	عصب	æ-SÆB
Nose	بینی	bee-NEE
Ovary	تخمدان	tokhm-DAN
Pancreas	لوزالمعده	lo-zol-me-DE
Penis	آلت	a-LÆT

Prostate	پروستات	pros-TAT
Rectum	مقعد	mæg-AD
Rib	دنده	dæn-DE
Shoulder	شانه	sha-NE
Skin	پوست	poost
Spleen	طحال	tæ-HAL
Spine	نخاع	no-KHA
Stomach	معده	me-DE
Teeth	دندانها	dæn-DAN-ha
Testicle	بیضه	bey-ZE
Throat	گلو	gæ-LOO
Thyroid	تیرویید	tee-ro-YEED
Toe	انگشت پا	æn-GOSH-te pa
Tonsils	لوزها	lo-ze-HA
Tongue	زبان	zæ-BAN
Uterus	رحم	ræ-HEM
Vagina	واژن	va-ZHÆN
Vein	ورید/سیاهرگ	væ-REED/see-yah-RÆG
Wrist	مچ	moch
NUMBERS		
How many (times)?	چند بار؟	chænd bar?
0	.	sef-r/heech
1	۱	yek
2	۲	do

(cont.)

3	۳	se
4	۴	cha-HAR
5	۵	pænj
6	۶	shesh
7	۷	hæft
8	۸	hæsh-t
9	۹	noh
10	۱۰	dæh
11	۱۱	yaz-DÆH
20	۲۰	beest
30	۳۰	see
40	۴۰	che-HEL
50	۵۰	pæn-JAH
60	۶۰	shæst
70	۷۰	hæf-TAD
80	۸۰	hæsh-TAD
90	۹۰	næ-VÆD
100	۱۰۰	SÆD

French—Français

WORD/PHRASE	TRANSLATION	ENGLISH PRONUNCIATION
French	Français	f-kha*ng*-SE

INTRODUCTION & REGISTRATION

Hello	Bonjour	bo*ng* ZHOO-kh
I am a doctor / nurse	Je suis médecin/ infirmière	zhu swee med-SE*ng*/ e*ng*-feekh-M-YE-khu
What is your name?	Comment vous appelez-vous ?	ku-MO*ng* vooz ap-LE VOO?
Who is your doctor?	Qui est votre médecin ?	kee VO-t-khe med-SE*ng*?
How old are you?	Quel âge avez-vous ?	kel azh a-ve-VOO?
Birthdate?	Date de naissance ?	dat du nE-SA*ng*-su?
Telephone number?	Numéro de téléphone ?	nü-me-KHO du te-le-FUN?
Address?	Adresse ?	ad-KHE-su?
Social security number?	Numéro de sécurité sociale ?	nü-me-KHO du se-kyü-khee-TE du so-S-YAL?
Insurance?	Assurance	a-sü-KHA*ng*-su

BASICS

Do you understand?	Comprenez-vous ?	kum-p-khu-ne VOO?
Yes	Oui	wee
No	Non	NO*ng*
Please	S'il vous plaît	seel voo PLE
Thank you	Merci	mekh-SEE
Sorry	Pardon	pakh-DO*ng*
I don't understand	Je ne comprends pas	zhu ne kum-p-KHA*ng* PA
Repeat	Répétez	khe-pe-TE

(cont.)

Speak slowly	Parlez lentement	pakh-LE lang-te-MAng
Answer "yes" or "no"	Répondez "oui" ou "non"	khe-pong-DE 'wee' oo 'nong'
Here	Ici	ee-SEE
This	Ceci	su-SEE
It's alright (consoling)	Tout va bien	TOO va b-YEng
I'll be right back	Je reviens tout de suite	zhu khu-vYEng to du SWEE-tu
GENERAL		
What's wrong?	Qu'est-ce qui ne va pas ?	KES kee nu va PA?
Pain	Douleur	doo-LUKH
Do you have pain?	Avez-vous mal ?	a-ve-VOO mal?
Does the pain radiate?	Est-ce que le mal se propage?	es ku lu MAL se p-kho-PAZH?
Where (show me)	Où (montrez moi)	OO (mong-T-KHE-MWA)
Gone now	C'est passé	sey pa-SE
Still present	Toujour là	too-ZHOOKH LA
Sudden/gradual onset	Commencement soudain/graduel	ku-mang-s-MAng soo-DEng/g-kha-dü-EL
What bothers you the most?	Qu'est-ce qui vous gêne le plus ?	KES kee voo zhen lu PLÜ?
Why did you come today?	Pour quelle raison êtes-vous venu aujourd'hui ?	pookh KEL khay-ZOng et voo vu-NÜ o-zhookh-DWEE
QUALITY		
If '0' is no pain and 10 is maximum pain, what number do you have now?	Si le numéro "zéro" est sans douleur et "dix" est la douleur maximum, quel numéro avez-vous maintenant ?	see lu nü-me- 'ze-KHO' e sang doo-LUKH e 'DEES' E la doo-LUKH mak-see-MUM, kel nü-me-KHO a-VE voo mEng-tu-nang

Burning	Brûlante	b-khü-La*ng*-tu
Constant	Constante	ko*ng*-STA*ng*T
Dull	Sourde	sookh-du
Intermittent	Intermittente	e*ng*-tekh-mee-TA*ng*T
Pressure	Pression	p-khe-S-YO*ng*
Severe	Sévère	se-VE-khu
Sharp/prickly pains	Aiguë/piquante	e-GÜ/pee-KA*ng*T
Throbbing	Lancinante	lang-see-NA*ng*T
ASSOCIATED SYMPTOMS		
Onset during... (before/after)	Qu'est-ce que vous faisez quand ceci a commencé? (avant/après)	KES ku voo fu-ZE ka*ng* se-SEE a ko-ma*ng*-SE
Worse (with...)	Est pire (avec...)	e PEE-khu (a-VEK...)
Better (with...)	Est meilleure (avec...)	e mey-YUKH (a-VEK...)
Cough	Toux	too
Deep breath	Respiration profonde	khu-spee-kha-S-YO*ng* p-kho-FO*ng*-du
Emotional upset	Bouleversé	bool-vekh-SE
Food	Nourriture	noo-khee-TYÜ-khu
Movement	Mouvement	moov-MA*ng*
Nothing	Rien	khee-E*ng*
Positioning	Position	po-zee-S-YO*ng*
Rest	Repos	re-PO
Walking	En marchant	ang makh-SHA*ng*
TIME COURSE		
For how long?	Pendant combien de temps ?	pa*ng*-DA*ng* kong-B-YE*ng* du TA*ng*?

(cont.)

Today	Aujourd'hui	o-zhookh-DWEE
Yesterday	Hier	ee-YE-kh
How many...	Combien de...?	ko*ng*-b-YE*ng* du...?
Months/weeks/days/hours/seconds	Mois/semaines/jours/heures/secondes	mwa/su-MEN/ZHOO-kh/U-kh/se-GO*ng*-du
Still present?	Toujours là ?	too-ZHOO-kh LA?
Gone now?	C'est passé ?	se pa-SE?
How long did it last? (See Number List)	Combien de temps cela a-t-il duré ?	co*ng*-b-YE*ng* de TA*ng* su-LA A-teel dyü-KHE?
Have you had this before?	Est-ce que vous avez déjà eu ça avant ?	es ku voo a-ve de-zha Ü sa a-VA*ng*?
How many times?	Combien de fois ?	ko*ng*-b-YE*ng* du F-WA?
When was the last time?	Quand a été la dernière fois?	ka*ng* A e-TE la dekh-N-YE-kh F-WA?
New	Nouveau	noo-VO
Old	Ancien	a*ng*-S-YE*ng*
CONTEXT		
Did you...?	Est-ce que vous...?	es ku voo...?
fall	êtes tombé ?	et to*ng*-BE?
trip	avez trébuché ?	voo za-ve tre-bü-SHE?
faint	vous vous êtes évanoui ?	voo vooz et e-va-noo-WEE?
twist	vous vous êtes foulé?	voo-voo zet foo-LE?
get hit	avez été heurté ?	vooz a-VEZ e-TE ukh-TE?
get burned	vous êtes brûlé ?	vooz et b-khü-LE?
get assaulted	avez été agressé ?	voo za-VE e-TE ag-khe-SE?
get bitten (human/dog/cat/insect)	avez été mordu ?	a-VEZ e-TE mor-DÜ?

French—Français

PAST MEDICAL HISTORY		
Take medication?	Prenez-vous des médicaments ?	p-khu-NE VOO dü me-dee-ka-MA*ng*?
(aspirin/antibiotics)	(aspirine/antibiotiques)	as-pee-KHEE-nu / a*ng*-tee-bee-o-TEE-ku
Do you have (See also Medical Problem List)…	Avez-vous…	a-ve VOO…
allergies	des allergies	dez a-lekh-ZHEE
medical problems	des problèmes médicaux	dey p-kho-BLEM me-dee-KO
Do you have problems of the… (see Body Parts List)	Avez-vous des problèmes de…	a-ve VOO de p-kho-BLEM du…
SURGICAL HISTORY		
Have you had surgery?	Avez-vous eu des opérations chirurgicales ?	a-ve-vooz-U dez-o-pe-kha-S-YO*ng* shee-khü-zhee-KA-lu?
Surgery on/"to remove"…(see Body Parts List)	Chirurgie de …	shee-khü-GEE du…
SOCIAL HISTORY		
Smoke?	Fumez-vous ?	fü-ME voo?
Drink?	Buvez-vous de l'alcool ?	bü-VE voo du lal-KOL?
Take drugs?	Prenez-vous de la drogue ?	p-khu-NE voo du la d-kho-gu?
Recent travel?	Voyage recent ?	v-way-AZH re-SA*ng*?
Are you sexually active?	Avezvous des relations sexuelles ?	a-ve-VOO de khu-la-S-YO*ng* sek-sü-EL?

(cont.)

Do you use condoms?	Utilisez-vous des préservatifs ?	ü-tee-lee-ze-VOO de p-ke-zekh-va-TEEF?
Homosexual	Homosexuel	o-mo-SEK-sü-EL

SYSTEMS REVIEW

Do you have...	Avez-vous...	a-ve-VOO...

GENERAL

Fever	Fièvre	F-YEV-khu
Chills	Frissons	f-khee-ZO*ng*
Weight loss	Perte de poids	PEKH-tu du PWA
Fatigue	Fatigue	fa-TEE-gu
Sick contact	Contact avec des malades	ko*ng*-TAK-T a-VEK de ma-LA-du

HEENT

Sore throat	Mal à la gorge	mal a la GOKH-zhu
Runny nose	Nez qui coule	ne kee KOO-lu
Nosebleed	Saignement du nez	se-nyu-MA*ng* dü ne
Ear pain	Mal à l'oreille	mal a lo-KHE-yu
Ear ringing	Bruits dans l'oreille	b-kh-WEE da*ng* lo-KHE-yu
Decreased hearing	Perte de l'ouïe	PEKH-tu du L-WEE

EYE

Eye pain	Mal aux yeux	mal o Z-YU
Blurry vision	Vue floue	vü f-loo
Diplopia	Diplopie / vision dédoublée	dee-plo-PEE / vee-ZYO*ng* DE-doob-LE
Foreign body sensation	Sensation d'un corps étranger	sa*ng*-sa-S-YO*ng* du*ng* KO-kh e-t-kha*ng*-ZHE
Contact lenses	Lentilles de contact	la*ng*-TEEY du ko*ng*-TAK-T

CARDIAC		
Chest pain	Mal à la poitrine	mal a la pwa-T-KHEE-nu
Palpitations	Palpitations	pal-pee-ta-S-YO*ng*
Orthopnea	Orthopnée (Difficulté à respirer quand vous êtes allongé à plat)	okh-top-NE (dee-fee-kül-TE a res-pee-RE ko*ng* vooz ET a-lo*ng*-ZHE a PLA)
Dyspnea on exertion	Essoufflement lors d'un exercice physique	e-soo-flu-MA*ng* lokh dun ek-zer-SEES
Fainting (syncope)	Évanouissement	e-va-noo-ee-su-Ma*ng*
Leg swelling	Enflure de la jambe	a*ng*-FLÜ-khu du la ZHA*ng*-bu
How many pillows?	Combien d'oreillers?	ko*ng*-b-YE*ng* do-khe-YE ?
PULMONARY		
Trouble breathing	Difficulté à respirer	dee-fee-kül-TE a khe-spee-KHE
SOB	Essoufflement	e-soo-flu-MA*ng*
Cough	Toux	too
Sputum	Expectoration	ek-spek-to-kha-S-YO*ng*
Pain on inspiration	Mal à l'inspiration	mal a le*ng*-spee-kha-S-YO*ng*
Hemoptysis	Crachement de sang	k-khash-MA*ng* du Sa*ng*
GI		
Abdominal pain	Douleur abdominale	doo-LUKH ab-do-mee-NA-lu
Nausea	Nausée	no-ZE
Vomiting	Vomissement	vo-mee-su-MA*ng*
Vomiting blood	Vomissement de sang	vo-mees-MO*ng* du SA*ng*
Coffee ground emesis	Vomissement ressemblant à de la mouture de café	vo-mees-MO*ng* ru-sem-BLA*ng* A du la moo-TÜKH du ka-FE

(cont.)

Anorexia	Anorexie	a-no-rek-SEE
Diarrhea	Diarrhée	d-ya-KHE
Difficulty swallowing	Difficulté à avaler	dee-fee-kül-TE a a-va-LE
BRBPR	La selle sanglante	la sel sa*ng*-GLA*ng*-tu
Melena	La selle noire	la sel NWA-khu
Pain after eating	Douleur après avoir mangé	doo-LUKH a-P-KHES a-V-WA-kh ma*ng*-ZHE
Worms	Vers	VE-kh
Constipation	Constipation	ko*ng*-stee-pa-S-YO*ng*
GU		
Painful urination	Urination douleureuse	ü-khee-na-S-YO*ng* doo-lu-KHU-zu
Urgent urination	Urination pressante	ü-khee-na-S-YO*ng* p-khe-SA*ng*-tu
Frequent urination	Urination fréquente	ü-khee-na-S-YO*ng* f-khe-KA*ng*-tu
Bloody urination	Urination contenant du sang	ü-khee-na-S-YO*ng* ko*ng*-tu-NA*ng* dü SA*ng*
Discharge: vaginal/penile	Décharge: vaginal/du pénis	de-SHAKH-zhe: va-zhee-NA-lu/dü pe-NEES
PSYCH		
Anxiety	Angoisse	a*ng*-GWAS
Depression	Dépression	de-p-khe-S-YO*ng*
Suicidal thoughts	Pensées suicidaires	pa*ng*-SE swee-see-DE-khu
Homicidal thoughts	Pensées homicides	pa*ng*-SE o-mee-SEE-du
Medication overdose	Surdose de médicaments	sookh-DOZ du me-dee-ka-MA*ng*
Hear voices	Entendez-vous des voix	a*ng*-TA*ng*-de voo du v-wa

NEURO		
Headache	Mal à la tête	mal a la TET
Worst headache of life	Le pire mal de tête de votre vie	lu PEER mal du TET du vot-khe VEE
Weakness	Faiblesse	fe-BLE-su
Dizzy	Pris de vertige	p-khee du vekh-TEE-zhu
What is your name?	Comment vous appellez-vous ?	ku-MO*ng* vooz a-pu-le-VOO ?
Where are we?	Où sommes nous ?	oo sum NOO ?
What is the year/month/date?	Quel est l'année/le mois/la date ?	KEL e la-NE/lu mwa/la DA-tu ?
Bowel dysfunction	Problèmes au niveau des gros intestins	p-khob-LEM O nee-VO de g-kho zeng-tes-TE*ng*
Bladder dysfunction	Problèmes au niveau de la vessie	p-khob-LEM O nee-VO de du la ve-SEE
Photophobia	Photophobie (sensibilité à la lumière)	fo-to-fo-BEE (seng-see-bee-lee-TE a la lüm-YE-khu)
Tingling/numbness	Picotement/engourdissement	pee-KO-tu-MA*ng*/a*ng*-gookh-dee-su-MA*ng*
Decreased strength in…(See Body Part List)	Force diminuée dans…	FOKH-su dee-mee-nü-E da*ng*…
Seizure	Convulsion	co*ng*-vül-Z-YO*ng*
Difficulty walking	Difficulté à marcher	dee-fee-kül-TE a makh-SHE
Difficulty speaking	Difficulté à parler	dee-fee-kül-TE a pakh-LE
Spinning (vertigo)	Étourdissement (vertige)	e-tookh-dee-su-MA*ng* (vekh-TEE-zhu)
Confusion	Confusion	ko*ng*-fü-ZYO*ng*

(cont.)

MISC		
Lump	Boule	BOO-lu
Itching	Démangeaison	de-mang-zhe-ZOng
Bruising	Contusions	kong-tü-Z-YOng
Rash	Éruption cutanée	e-khüp-S-YOng k-yü-ta-NE
Swelling	Enflure	ang-FLÜ-khu
Jaundice (yellow skin)	Jaunisse	zho-NEE-su
GYNECOLOGIC		
Vaginal bleeding	Saignement vaginal	se-nyu-MAng va-zhee-NAL
Heavy	Intense, excessif	eng-TAng-su, ek-se-SEEF
Irregular	Irrégulier	EE-khe-gü-L-YE
Absent	Absent	ab-SAng
Vaginal discharge	Décharge vaginale	de-SHAKH-zhu va-zhee-NA-lu
Pelvic pain	Douleur au pelvis	doo-LUKH o pel-VEES
Rape	Viol	vee-OL
Pain with intercourse	Douleur durant les rapports sexuels	doo-LUKH dü-KHAng le kha-POKH sek-soo-EL
Contraceptive	Contraceptif	kong-t-kha-sep-TEEF
OBSTETRIC		
Are you pregnant?	Est-ce que vous êtes enceinte?	es ku voos et ang-SEng-tu
LMP how many days ago?	Quand avez-vous eu vos dernières règles ?	kang a-ve-VOO ü vo dekh-N-YE KHEG-lu?
Times pregnant?	Combien de fois avez-vous été enceinte ?	kong-b-YEng de fwa a-ve vooz e-TE ang-SEng-tu?

Times delivered?	Combien de fois avez-vous accouché ?	ko*ng*-b-YE*ng* de fwa a-VE voo a-koo-SHE?
Miscarriage	Perte du bébé	PEKH-tu dü be-BE
Abortion	Avortement	a-vokh-tu-MA*ng*
Fluid leakage	Fuite du sac d'eau	F-WEE-tu dü sak do
Contraction	Contraction	ko*ng*-t-khak-S-YO*ng*
Fetal movement	Mouvement du foetus	moo-vu-MA*ng* dü fe-TUS
TRAUMA		
How many hours ago did you eat last?	Quand avez-vous mangé la dernière fois ?	ka*ng* a-VE voo ma*ng*-ZHE la dekh-NYEKH f-WA?
Lost consciousness?	Perte de connaissance ?	PEKH-tu du ku-ne-SA*ng*-su
Tetanus within 5 years?	Tétanos dans les 5 dernières années ?	te-ta-NOS da*ng* le SE*ng*-k dekh-n-YE-khu a-NE?
PEDIATRIC		
How old?	Quel âge ?	kel A-zhu?
Vaccines up to date?	Vaccinations à jour ?	vak-see-na-S-YO*ng* a zhoo-kh?
Urinating normally	Urinez normallement	ü-khee-NE nokh-mal-MA*ng*
Taking liquids	Prise de boissons liquides	p-KHEES du b-wa-SO*ng* lee-KEE-du
Increased crying	Pleurs de plus en plus fréquents	plu-KHE du plü za*ng* plü f-khe-KA*ng*
Ingestion	Ingestion	e*ng*-jes-T-YO*ng*
Foreign body	Corps étranger	ko-kh e-t-kha*ng*-GE
Premature	Prématuré	p-khe-ma-t-yü-KHE
Birth complications	Complications à la naissance	ko*ng*-plee-ka-S-YO*ng* a la e-SA*ng*-su

(cont.)

PHYSICAL EXAM/INSTRUCTION		
Sit down (please)	Asseyez-vous (s'il vous plaît)	a-se-ye voo (seel voo ple)
Lie down	Allongez-vous	a-long-zhe-voo
Come here	Venez ici	vu-NE zee-SEE
Relax	Détendez-vous	DE-tang-de-VOO
Don't move	Ne bougez pas	ne boo-zhe PA
Open your mouth	Ouvrez la bouche	oo-V-KHE la BOO-shu
Say "ahh"	Dites "ahh"	deet "a"
Swallow	Avalez	a-va-LE
Breath deeply	Respirez profondément	khes-pee-KHE p-kho-fong-du-MAng
Hold your breath	Retenez votre souffle	ru-tu-NE VOT-khu SOO-flu
Cough	Toussez	too-SE
Push	Poussez	poo-SE
Pull	Tirez	tee-KHE
Follow my finger	Suivez mon doigt	s-wee-VE mong d-wa
Close your eyes	Fermez les yeux	fekh-ME lez YU
Smile	Souriez	soo-khee-YE
Can you feel this?	Sentez-vous ceci ?	sang-te-VOO se-SEE ?
Copy this (movement)	Copiez-moi (mouvement)	ko-pee-YE m-wa
I am going to put a finger in your rectum	Je vais mettre mon doigt dans votre rectum	zhu ve MET-khu mong dwa dang VOT-khu khek-TÜM
I am going to examine your vagina	Je vais examiner votre vagin	zhu ve ek-za-mee-NE VOT-khu va-ZHEng
REASSESSMENT		
Do you feel better?	Vous sentez-vous mieux ?	voo sang-te-VOO m-YU?

Do you feel worse?	Vous sentez-vous moins bien ?	voo sa*ng*-te-VOO m-WA*ng* b-YE*ng*?
PATIENT WORDS		
I hurt	J'ai mal	zhe mal
Help!	Au secours !	o su-KOO-kh!
Bathroom	Toilettes	t-wa-LET-tu
Food	Nourriture	noo-khee-TYÜ-khu
Water	Eau	o
PROCEDURES & CONSENT		
You need...	Vous avez besoin de...	voos a-VE bu-Z-WE*ng* du
Injection	Une injection	Ü-nu e*ng*-jek-S-YO*ng*
Stiches	Points de suture	p-WÆ du soo-TYÜ-khu
Cast	Plâtre	PLAT-khu
Crutches	Béquilles	be-KEE-yu
Perform surgery on the... (See Body Part List)	Opération chirurgicale	o-pe-kha-S-YO*ng* shee-khü-zhee-KA-lu
The risks are...	Les dangers sont...	le da*ng*-ZHE so*ng*...
Bleeding	Saignement	se-n-yu-MA*ng*
Infection	Infection	e*ng*-fek-S-YO*ng*
Scar	Cicatrice	see-ka-T-KHEE-su
Repeat procedure	Répéter la procédure	re-pe-TE la p-kho-se-D-YÜ-khu
Iodine	Iode	ee-O-du
Damage to your... (See Body Part List)	Blessure	ble-SYÜ-khu
Sign here	Signez ici	see-N-YE ee-SEE

(cont.)

TESTS		
X-ray	Radiographie	kha-dee-o-g-kha-FEE
C.A.T. Scan	Tomodensitogramme	to-mo-DA*ng*-see-to-g-KHAM
Ultrasound	Ultrason / échographie	ül-t-kha-SO*ng*/ e-ko-g-kha-FEE
Catheterization/ bladder catheter	Cathetirisation / catheter vesical	ka-te-tee-khee-za-S-YO*ng*/ka-te-TE-kh ve-see-KAL
Colonoscopy (from below)/Endoscopy (from above)	Colonoscopie	ko-lo-no-sko-PEE
Endoscopy	Endoscopie	a*ng*-do-sko-PEE
END OF LIFE		
Do you want us to…	Voulez-vous que nous…	voo-le-VOO ke noo…
Perform CPR	ferions réanimation cardio-respiratoire	fe-khee-YO*ng* khe-a-nee-ma-SYO*ng*/ kakh-dee-o-khes-peekh-at-WAkh
Defibrillate	ferions défibrillation	fe-khee-YO*ng* de-fee-b-ree-LE
Intubate	ferions insertion d'un tube	Fe-khee-YO*ng* e*ng*-se-KHE ung TÜ-bu
He/she is dead	Il / Elle est mort(e)	eel / EL e MOKH(-tu)
We did all we could	On avait fait tout ce qu'on pouvait	o-na-ve FE too su ko*ng* poo-VE
DISCHARGE		
You have…(See Medical Prob List)	Vous avez…	vooz a-VE…
He/she is going to stay in the hospital	Il/elle va rester à l'hôpital	eel/E-lu va khes-TE a lo-pee-TAL
Take "X" pills "Y" times a day for "Z" days	Prenez "X" comprimés "Y" fois par jour pour "Z" jours	p-khu-NE "X" ko*ng*-p-khee-ME "Y" f-wa pakh zhookh pookh "Z" zhookh

Pills	Comprimés	ko*ng*-p-khee-ME
Antibiotics	Antibiotiques	a*ng*-tee-bee-o-TEEK
Before/after meals	Avant / Après le repas	a-VA*ng* / a-P-KHE lu khu-PA
Return to the ER if...	Retourner à l'urgence si	khu-tookh-NE a lükh-ZHA*ng*-su see
Follow up at "X" on "Y"	Rendez-vous à "X" le "Y"	kha*ng*-de-VOO a "X" lu "Y"
You're welcome	Je vous en prie	zhu VOOS a*ng* P-KHEE
Goodbye	Au revoir	o khuv-WA-kh
MEDICAL PROBS		
AIDS/HIV	SIDA / VIH	see-DA / ve-ee-ASH
Anemia	Anémie	a-ne-MEE
Arrhythmia	Arhythmie	a-kheet-MEE
Arthritis	Arthrite	akh-T-KHEE-tu
Asthma	Asthme	AS-mu
Bronchitis	Bronchite	b-kho*ng*-SHEE-tu
Cancer	Cancer	ka*ng*-SE-kh
Cirrhosis	Cirrhose	see-KHO-zu
Cholesterol	Cholestérol	ko-les-te-KHOL
Cold	Rhume	KHÜ-mu
Constipation	Constipation	ko*ng*-stee-pa-S-YO*ng*
Cyst	Cyste	SEES-tu
Diabetes	Diabète	dee-a-BET-tu
Dialysis	Dialyse	dee-a-LEE-zu
Diverticulitis	Diverticulite	dee-vekh-tee-k-yü-LEE-tu
Emphysema	Emphysème	a*ng*-fee-ZE-mu

(cont.)

Fibroids	Fibromes	feeb-KHO-mu
Fracture	Fracture	f-khak-tyü-khu
Flu	Grippe/influenza	g-KHEE-pu/eng-flü-ang-za
Gallstones	Calculs biliaires	Ka-KÜL bee-lee-E-khu
Gastritis/GERD	Gastrite/reflux gastro-œsophagien	gas-T-KHEE-tu / khu-FLÜ gas-t-KHO e-so-fa-ZHYEng
Hepatitis	Hépatite	e-pa-TEE-tu
Heart attack	Crise cardiaque	k-KHEE-su kakh-dee-AK
Heart disease	Maladie du cœur	ma-la-DEE dü KU-kh
Heart failure	Affaiblissement du coeur	a-fe-blees-MAng dü KE-kh
Hypertension	Hypertension	ee-pekh-tang-S-YOng
Indigestion	Indigestion	eng-dee-jes-T-YOng
Kidney stone	Pierres dans les reins	PYE-khu dang le KHEng
Lupus	Lupus	loo-POOS
Migraine	Migraine	meeg-KHEN
Murmur	Souffle au cœur	SOOF-lu o KU-kh
Pacemaker	Stimulateur cardiaque	stee-m-yü-la-TUKH kakh-dee-AK
Pneumonia	Pneumonie	nü-mo-NEE
Seizures	Convulsions	kong-vül-Z-YOng
STD	Maladie vénérienne	ma-la-DEE ve-ne-khee-E-nu
Stroke	Accident cérébrovas-culaire	ak-see-DAng se-ke-b-kho-vas-kü-LEKH
Ulcer	Ulcère	ül-SEKH
Ulcerative colitis	Inflammation du colon / Colite ulcéreuse	eng-fla-ma-S-YOng dü ko-Long / ko-LEET ül-sekh-uz

French—Français

UTI	Infection urinaire	eng-fek-S-YOng ü-khee-NE-khu
BODY PARTS		
Abdomen	L'abdomen	lab-do-MEN
Ankle	La cheville	la shu-VEE-yu
Appendix	L'appendice	la-peng-DEE-su
Arm	Le bras	lu b-kha
Artery	L'artère	lakh-TE-khu
Back	Le dos	lu do
Bladder	La vessie	la ve-SEE
Blood	Le sang	lu sang
Bone	L'os	los
Brain	Le cerveau	lu sekh-VO
Breast	Le sein	lu seng
Calf	Le mollet	lu mo-LE
Chest	La poitrine	la p-wa-T-KHEE-nu
Chin	Le menton	lu mang-TOng
Ear	L'oreille	lo-KHE-yu
Elbow	Le coude	lu KOO-du
Eye	L'œil	LUY
Face	La figure	la fee-G-YÜ-khu
Finger	Le doigt	lu d-wa
Foot	Le pied	lu p-YE
Hand	La main	la meng
Head	La tête	la TE-tu
Heart	Le cœur	la KU-kh

(cont.)

Gallbladder	La vésicule billiaire	la ve-zee-KÜ-lu bee-lee-E-khu
Jaw	La mâchoire	la ma-SH-WA-khu
Joint	L'articulation	lakh-tee-kü-la-S-YOng
Kidney	Le rein	lu kheng
Knee	Le genou	lu zhu-NOO
Leg	La jambe	la ZHAng-bu
Liver	Le foie	lu f-wa
Mouth	La bouche	la BOO-shu
Muscle	Le muscle	lu MÜS-k-lu
Neck	Le cou	lu koo
Nerve	Le nerf	lu NEKH-f
Nose	Le nez	lu ne
Ovary	L'ovaire	lo-VE-khu
Pancreas	Le pancréas	lu pang-k-khe-AS
Penis	Le pénis	lu pe-NEES
Prostate	La prostate	la p-khos-TA-tu
Rectum	Le rectum	lu khek-TÜM
Rib	La côte	la KOT
Shoulder	L'épaule	le-PO-lu
Skin	La peau	la po
Spleen	La rate	la KHA-tu
Spine	La colonne vertébrale	lu ko-LO-nu vekh-te-B-KHA-lu
Stomach	L'estomac	les-to-MAK
Teeth	Les dents	le DAng
Testicle	Le testicule	lu tes-tee-KÜ-lu
Throat	La gorge	la GOKH-zhu

Thyroid	Le thyroïde	lu tee-kho-EE-du
Toe	L'orteil	lokh-TE-yu
Tonsils	Les amygdales	le a-meeg-DA-lu
Tongue	La langue	la LAng-gu
Uterus	L' utérus	lü-te-RÜS
Vagina	Le vagin	lu va-ZHEng
Vein	La veine	la VE-nu
Wrist	Le poignet	lu p-wa-N-YE
NUMBERS		
How many (times)?	Combien (de fois) ?	kong-b-YEng (du f-wa) ?
0	Zéro	ze-KHO
1	Un	ung
2	Deux	du
3	Trois	t-kh-wa
4	Quatre	KAT-khu
5	Cinq	seng-k
6	Six	sees
7	Sept	set
8	Huite	WEE-tu
9	Neuf	nuf
10	Dix	dees
11	Onze	ong-zu
20	Vingt	veng
30	Trente	T-KHAng-tu
40	Quarante	ka-KHAng-tu
50	Cinquante	seng-KAng-tu

60	Soixante	s-wa-SA*ng*-tu
70	Soixante-dix	s-wa-sa*ng*-tu-DEES
80	Quatre-vingt	ka-t-khu-VE*ng*
90	Quatre-vingt-dix	ka-t-khu-ve*ng*-DEES
100	Cent	sa*ng*

German—Deutsch

WORD/PHRASE	TRANSLATION	ENGLISH PRONUNCIATION
German	Deutsch	DOYCH
INTRODUCTION & REGISTRATION		
Hello	Hallo	HA-lo
I am doctor (m/f) / nurse (f/m) *(add your name)*	Ich bin Dr.[name] / Krankenschwester (f) [name] / Krankenpfleger (m) [name]	eekh bin DOK-tor [...] / KRAN-ken-sh-vester [...] / KRANK-ken-fley-ger [...]
What is your name?	Wie heissen Sie?	vee HAYS-sen zee?
Who is your doctor?	Wer ist ihr Arzt?	ver ist eer ART-ST?
How old are you?	Wie alt sind Sie?	vee ALT zint zee?
Birthdate?	Geburtstag?	ge-BOORTS-tak?
Telephone number?	Telefonnummer?	TEY-le-fon NOOM-mer?
Address?	Adresse?	ad-DRES-se?
Social security number?	Sozialversicherungsnummer?	zo-tsee-AL-fer-ZEEKH-er-oong-z-NOOM-mer?
Insurance?	Krankenversicherung?	KRAN-ken-fer-ZEEKH-er-oonk?
BASICS		
Do you understand?	Verstehen Sie?	fer-SH-TEY-en zee?
Yes	Ja	YA
No	Nein	nayn
Please	Bitte	BI-te
Thank you	Danke	DAN-ke
Sorry	Entschuldigung	ent-SHOOL-dee-goong
I don't understand	Ich verstehe nicht	eekh fer-SHTEY-e neekh-t
Repeat	Wiederholen Sie	vee-der-HOL-en zee

(cont.)

Speak slowly	Langsam sprechen	LANG-zam sh-PRE-khen
Answer "yes" or "no"	Antworten Sie "ja" oder "nein"	ant-VORT-en zee YA O-der NAYN
Here	Hier	heer
This	Dies(e)	dees (dee-ze)
It's alright (consoling)	Es ist schon gut	es ist shon GOOT
I'll be right back	Ich komme gleich wieder	eekh KOM-me glaykh VEE-der
GENERAL		
What's wrong?	Was ist Loss?	vas ist LOS?
Pain	Schmerz	sh-MER-ts
Do you have pain?	Haben Sie Schmerzen?	HA-ben zee sh-MER-tsen?
Does the pain radiate?	Ist der Schmerz ausstrahlend?	ist der sh-MER-ts a-oos-STRA-lent?
Where (show me)	Zeigen Sie mir wo	TSAY-gen zee meer VO
Gone now	Im Moment nicht da	im mo-MENT neekh-t DA
Still present	Noch da	nokh da
Sudden/gradual onset	Plötzlicher/allmählicher Anfang	PLUTS-lee-kher / al-MEY-lee-kher AN-fang
What bothers you the most?	Was stört Sie am meisten?	vas sh-TERT zee am MAY-sten?
Why did you come today?	Warum sind Sie heute hergekommen?	va-ROOM zind zee HOY-te HER-ge-kom-men?
QUALITY		
If '0' is no pain and 10 is maximum pain, what number do you have now?	Wenn "0" schmerzlos ist, und 10 am schmerzhaftesten, wie beschreiben Sie Ihren Schmerz?	ven nool SHMER-ts-los ist, oond TSEYN am sh-MER-ts-haft-EST-en, vee be-SHREY-ben zee EE-ren sh-MER-ts?
Burning	Brennend	BREN-end
Constant	Konstant	kon-STANT

Dull	Dumpf	DOOM-f
Intermittent	Kommend und gehend	KOM-mend oony GEY-ent
Pressure	Druck	drook
Severe	Stark	sh-TAR-k
Sharp/prickly pains	Heftig / stechend	HEF-tik / SHTEY-khent
Throbbing	Pochend	PO-khend
ASSOCIATED SYMPTOMS		
Onset during... (before/after)	Anfang während... (for/nach)	AN-fang VEY-rend...
Worse (with...)	Schlimmer mit...	SH-LIM-mer mit...
Better (with...)	Besser mit...	BES-ser mit...
Cough	Husten	HOOS-ten
Deep breath	Beim tief Einatmen	baym TEEF ayn-AT-men
Emotional upset	Emotionelle Verstimmung	e-mo-tsee-O-NA-le ver-SH-TIM-moonk
Food	Essen	ES-sen
Movement	Bewegung	be-VEY-goong
Nothing	Nichts	nikh-ts
Positioning	Position	PO-zee-ts-YON
Rest	Ruhe	ROO-e
Walking	Gehen	GEY-en
TIME COURSE		
For how long?	Für wie lange?	für vee LAN-ge?
Today	Heute	HOY-te
Yesterday	Gestern	GES-tern
How many...	Wie viele...?	vee FEE-le?

(cont.)

Months/weeks/days/hours/seconds	Monate/Wochen/Tage/Stunden/Minuten/Sekunden	MO-na-te, VOKH-en, SH-TOON-den, mee-NOO-ten, zey-KOON-den
Still present?	Immer noch da?	IM-mer nokh da?
Gone now?	Jetzt weg?	yet-st veyk?
How long did it last? (See Numbers List)	Wie Lange hat es gedauert?	vee LAN-ge hat es ge-DOY-ert?
Have you had this before?	Hatten Sie so etwas schon einmal?	HAT-ten zee zo ET-vas shon AYN-mal?
How many times?	Wie viele Male?	vee FEE-le MA-le?
When was the last time?	Wann war das letzte Mal?	van var das LETS-te mal?
New	Neu	noy
Old	Alt	alt
CONTEXT		
Did you…?	Sind Sie…?	zint zee…?
fall	…gefallen?	ge-FAL-len?
trip	…gestolpert?	ge-SH-TOL-pert?
faint	…ohnmächtig geworden?	ON-meykh-tig ge-VORD-en?
twist	Haben Sie sich falsch gedreht?	HA-ben zee zeekh fal-SH ge-DREY-t?
get hit	Wurden Sie geschlagen?	VOORD-en zee ge-SH-LA-gen?
get burned	Haben Sie Sich verbrannt?	HA-ben zee sikh ver-BRAN-T?
get assaulted	Wurden Sie angegriffen?	VOORD-en zee an-ge-GRI-fen?
get bitten (human/dog/cat/insect)	Wurden Sie gebissen?	VOORD-en zee ge-BIS-sen

PAST MEDICAL HISTORY		
Take medication?	Nehmen Sie Medikamente?	NEY-men zee mey-dee-ka-MEN-te?
(aspirin/antibiotics)	Aspirin/Antibiotikum	ah-SPEY-reen / an-TEE-bee-YO-tee-koom
Do you have (See also Medical Problem List)...	Haben Sie...	HA-ben zee...
allergies	Allergien	al-ler-GEE-en
medical problems	Medizinische Probleme	me-dee-ZEEN-ish-e pro-BLEY-me
Do you have problems of the... (see Body Parts List)	Haben Sie Probleme mit...	HA-ben zee pro-BLEY-me mit...
SURGICAL HISTORY		
Have you had surgery?	Sind Sie schon mal operiert worden?	zind zee shon mal o-pa-REERT VOR-den?
Surgery on/"to remove"...(see Body Parts List)	Operation an ...	o-pa-ra-tsee-ON an
SOCIAL HISTORY		
Smoke?	Rauchen Sie?	RAU-khen zee
Drink?	Trinken Sie Alkohol?	TRIN-ken zee al-ko-HOL?
Take drugs?	Nehmen Sie Drogen?	NEY-men zee DRO-gen?
Recent travel?	Sind Sie in letzter Zeit verreist?	zind zee in LETS-ter TSAYT ver-RAYST?
Are you sexually active?	Sind Sie sexuell aktiv?	zind zee ZEKS-oo-el ak-TEEF?
Do you use condoms?	Benutzen Sie Kondome?	be-NOOTZ-en zee kon-DO-me?
Homosexual	Sind Sie homosexuell?	zint zee HO-mo-ZEKS-u-el?

(cont.)

SYSTEMS REVIEW		
Do you have…	Haben Sie…	HA-ben zee…
GENERAL		
Fever	Fieber	FEE-ber
Chills	Frösteln	FRES-tel-n
Weight loss	Gewicht verloren	ge-VIKHT ver-LOR-en
Fatigue	Müdigkeit	MÜ-dig-kayt
Sick contact	Kontakt mit einer kranken Person	kon-TAK-T mit AY-ner KRANK-en per-ZON
HEENT		
Sore throat	Halsschmerzen	HALS-SH-MERTS-en
Runny nose	Nasenlaufen	NA-zen-LAU-fen
Nosebleed	Nasenbluten	NA-zen-BLOO-ten
Ear pain	Ohrenschmerzen	OR-en-SH-MERTS-en
Ear ringing	Ohrensausen	OR-en-ZAU-zen
Decreased hearing	Hörverlust	HER-ver-loost
EYE		
Eye pain	Augenschmerzen	AU-gen-SH-MERTS-en
Blurry vision	Verschwommene Sicht	ver-SH-VOM-en-e sikh-t
Diplopia	Doppeltsehen	DOP-pelt-ZEY-en
Foreign body sensation	Gefühl der Anwesenheit eines Fremdkörpers	ge-FÜL der an-VEY-zen-hayt AY-nes FREM-D-ker-pers
Contact lenses	Kontaktlinsen	KON-takt-LIN-zen
CARDIAC		
Chest pain	Brustschmerz	BROOST-sh-merts
Palpitations	Herzklopfen	HERTS-klopf-en
Orthopnea	Atemnot beim Liegen (Orthopnoe)	A-tem-not baym LEE-gen (or-TOP-noe)

Dyspnea on exertion	Atemnot bei Belastung (Dyspnoe)	A-tem-not bay be-LAS-toonk (DOOSP-no-e)
Fainting (syncope)	Ohnmacht (Synkope)	ON-makht (ZOON-ko-pe)
Leg swelling	Angeschwollene Beine	an-ge-sh-VOL-len-e BEY-ne
How many pillows?	Wie viele Kopfkissen?	vee FEE-le KOF-kis-sen?
PULMONARY		
Trouble breathing	Schweres Atmen	SHVEY-res AT-men
SOB	Atemnot	A-tem-NOT
Cough	Husten	HOO-sten
Sputum	Sputum	SH-POO-tum
Pain on inspiration	Schmerz beim Einatmen	sh-MERTS baym AYN-at-men
Hemoptysis	Blutiger Auswurf	BLOO-ti-ger AOS-voorf
GI		
Abdominal pain	Bauchschmerzen	BAUKH-shmeyr-tsen
Nausea	Übelkeit	Ü-bel-kayt
Vomiting	Erbrechen	ER-bre-khen
Vomiting blood	Blutige Übergebung	BLOO-tee-ge Ü-ber-GEY-boong
Coffee ground emesis	Kaffeesatzerbrechen (schwarzes Erbrechen)	KAF-fey-zats-ER-brekh-en (sh-VAR-tses ER-bre-khen)
Anorexia	Magersucht	MA-ger-sookh-t
Diarrhea	Diarrhea / Durchfall	DEE-ah-REY-ah / DOORKH-fal
Difficulty swallowing	Beschwerden beim Schlucken	be-sh-VER-den baym sh-LOO-ken
BRBPR	Helles rotes Blut pro Mastdarm	HEL-les RO-tes BLOOT pro MAST-darm

(cont.)

Melena	Melena	MEY-LE-na
Pain after eating	Schmerzen nach dem Essen	SH-MERTS-en nakh deym ES-sen
Worms	Würmer	VÜR-mer
Constipation	Verstopfung	fer-SH-TOP-foong
GU		
Painful urination	Schmerzhaftes Urinieren	SH-MERTS-haf-tes o-REE-NEE-ren
Urgent urination	Harndrang	HARN-drank
Frequent urination	Häufiges Urinieren	HOY-fee-ges o-REE-NEE-ren
Bloody urination	Blut im Harn	bloot im harn
Discharge: vaginal/penile	Ausfluss: Scheide / Penis	AUS-floos: SHAY-de / PEY-nis
PSYCH		
Anxiety	Angstzustände	ang-st-tsoo-sh-TEN-de
Depression	Depressionen	dey-pres-zee-O-nen
Suicidal thoughts	Selbstmordgedanken	zelb-st-mord-ge-DAN-ken
Homicidal thoughts	Mordgedanken	MORD-ge-DANK-ken
Medication overdose	Arzneimittelüberdosis	arts-NAY-MIT-tel-ü-ber-DO-sis
Hear voices	Höhren Sie Stimmen?	HU-ren zee sh-TIM-men?
NEURO		
Headache	Kopfschmerzen	kop-f-SH-MERTS-en
Worst headache of life	Die schlimmsten Kopfschmerzen des Lebens	dee SH-LIM-sten kop-f-SH-MERTS-en des LEY-bens
Weakness	Schwäche	SH-VE-khe
Dizzy	Schwindlig	SH-VIND-leeg

What is your name?	Wie heissen Sie?	vee HAY-sen zee?
Where are we?	Wo sind wir?	VO zint veer?
What is the year/month/date?	Was ist das Jahr/Monat/Datum?	vas ist das yahr / MO-nat / DA-tum
Bowel dysfunction	Darmstörung	darm-sh-TER-roong
Bladder dysfunction	Blasenstörung	BLA-zen-STER-roong
Photophobia	Abnomale Lichtempfindlichkeit	ab-nor-MAL-e leekh-tem-FINDK-leekh-kayt
Tingling/numbness	Kribbeln/Benommenheit	KRIB-bel-n/BEY-nom-men-hayt
Decreased strength in…(See Body Parts List)	Verminderte Kraft in…	fer-MIN-dert-e KRAFT in…
Seizure	Krampfanfall	KRAM-fan-fal
Difficulty walking	Schwierigkeiten beim Laufen	sh-VEE-rig-kayt-en baym LAU-fen
Difficulty speaking	Schwierigkeiten beim Reden	sh-VEE-rig-kayt-en baym REY-den
Spinning (vertigo)	Es dreht sich alles (Höhenschwindel)	es dreyt zeekh AL-les (HE-en-sh-VIN-del)
Confusion	Verwirrung	fer-VIR-roong
MISC		
Lump	Knoten / Beule	K-NO-ten / BOY-le
Itching	Jucken	YOO-ken
Bruising	Prellung	PREL-oong
Rash	Ausschlag	AUS-sh-lag
Swelling	Schwellung	SH-VEL-loong
Jaundice (yellow skin)	Gelbsucht	gel-b-ZOOKH-T

(cont.)

GYNECOLOGIC		
Vaginal bleeding	Vaginalblutung	va-gee-NAL-BLOO-toong
Heavy	Schwer	SH-VEYR
Irregular	Unregelmäßig	oon-RE-GEL-may-zeeg
Absent	Fehlt	fayl-t
Vaginal discharge	Scheidenausfluss	SHAY-den-AUS-flus
Pelvic pain	Beckenschmerz	BEK-en-sh-merts
Rape	Vergewaltigung	fer-GE-val-TEE-goong
Pain with intercourse	Schmerzen wärend des Geschlechtsverkehrs	SH-MERTS-en VEY-rend des ge-SH-LEKH-ts-FER-kers
Contraceptive	Verhütungsmittel	fer-HÜ-toongs-MIT-tel
OBSTETRIC		
Are you pregnant?	Sind Sie schwanger?	zint zee SH-VANG-er?
LMP how many days ago?	Vor wievielen Tagen hatten Sie zum letzten Mal Ihre Periode?	for vee-FEE-len Tag-en HAT-ten zee tsoom LET-tsen mal EE-re pe-ree-O-de?
Times pregnant?	Wie oft waren Sie schwanger?	vee OF-T VA-ren zee SH-VAN-ger?
Times delivered?	Wie viele Schwangerschaften haben Sie ausgetragen?	vee FEE-le SH-VAN-ger-SHAFT-en HA-ben zee AUS-ge-TRAG-en?
Miscarriage	Fehlgeburt	feyl-ge-BOORT
Abortion	Abtreibung	ap-TRAY-boong
Fluid leakage	Auslaufende Flüssigkeit	aus-LAU-fen-de FLOO-zeeg-kayt
Contraction	Wehen	VEY-en
Fetal movement	Fötale Bewegung	fu-TAL-e be-VEY-goong

German—Deutsch 71

TRAUMA		
How many hours ago did you eat last?	Vor wievielen Stunden haben Sie zuletzt gegessen?	for vee FEE-len SH-TOON-den HA-ben zee tsoo-LET-ST ge-GES-sen?
Lost consciousness?	Haben Sie das Bewusstsein verloren?	HA-ben zee das bey-VOOST-tseyn fer-LO-ren?
Tetanus within 5 years?	Hatten Sie in den letzten 5 Jahren eine Tetanusimpfung?	HAT-ten zee in den LETS-ten funf YA-ren AY-ne TEY-ta-noos-im-foong?

PEDIATRIC		
How old?	Wie alt?	vee ALT?
Vaccines up to date?	Sind Ihre Impfungen auf dem letzten Stand?	zint EE-ra IMP-foong-en auf daym LETS-ten sh-TANT?
Urinating normally	Normales Wasserlassen	nor-MAL-es VAS-ser-LAS-sen
Taking liquids	Flüssigkeitenaufnahme	FLÜS-zeeg-kay-ten-AUF-NA-me
Increased crying	Übermäßiges Weinen	Ü-ber-MEY-see-ges VAY-nen
Ingestion	Einnahme	AYN-na-me
Foreign body	Fremdkörper	FREMT-ker-per
Premature	Frühgeburt	FRÜ-ge-boort
Birth complications	Komplikationen bei der Geburt	kom-PLEE-ka-tsee-O-nen bay der ge-BOORT

PHYSICAL EXAM/INSTRUCTION		
Sit down (please)	Setzen Sie sich (bitte)	ZETS-en zee sikh (BIT-te)
Lie down	Liegen Sie sich hin	LEE-gen zee sikh hin
Come here	Kommen Sie her	KOM-men zee her
Relax	Entspannen Sie sich	ent-SH-PAN-en zee sikh

(cont.)

72 German—Deutsch

Don't move	Halten Sie still	HAL-ten zee sh-til
Open your mouth	Öffnen Sie den Mund	UF-nen zee den moond
Say "ahh"	Sagen Sie "ahh"	ZA-gen zee "ah"
Swallow	Schlucken Sie	SH-LOOK-en zee
Breath deeply	Atmen Sie tief durch	AT-men zee TEEF doorkh
Hold your breath	Halten Sie den Atem an	HAL-ten zee deyn A-tem an
Cough	Husten Sie	HOOST-en zee
Push	Pressen (Drucken) Sie	PRES-sen (DROOK-en) zee
Pull	Ziehen Sie	TSEE-en zee
Follow my finger	Folgen Sie meinem Finger	FOL-gen zee MAY-nem FIN-ger
Close your eyes	Schließen Sie die Augen	SH-LEE-sen zee dee AU-gen
Smile	Lächeln Sie	LEKH-el-n zee
Can you feel this?	Spüren Sie dies?	SH-PÜ-ren zee dees?
Copy this (movement)	Machen Sie diese (Bewegung) nach	MA-khen zee dee-ze (be-VEY-goong) nakh
I am going to put a finger in your rectum	Ich werde einen Finger in Ihrem Darm einführen	ikh VER-de AYN-en FING-er in EE-ren darm AYN-fü-ren
I am going to examine your vagina	Ich werde Ihre Scheide untersuchen	ikh VER-de EE-re SHAY-de oon-ter-ZOO-khen
REASSESSMENT		
Do you feel better?	Fühlen Sie sich besser?	FÜ-len zee sikh BES-ser?
Do you feel worse?	Fühlen Sie sich schlechter?	FÜ-len zee sikh SH-LEKH-ter?
PATIENT WORDS		
I hurt	Ich habe Schmerzen	ikh HA-be SH-MERTS-en
Help!	Hilfe!	HIL-fe!

German—Deutsch

Bathroom	Toilette / WC	TOY-let-te / VEY TSEY
Food	Essen	ES-sen
Water	Wasser	VAS-ser
PROCEDURES & CONSENT		
You need...	Sie brauchen...	zee BRAU-khen...
Injection	Eine Spritze	AY-ne sh-PRIT-tse
Stiches	Nähte	NEY-te
Cast	Gipsverband	GIPS-fer-BANT
Crutches	Stützen	sh-TÜ-tsen
Perform surgery on the... (See Body Parts List)	Operation an	o-per-a-tsee-ON an...
The risks are...	Die Risiken sind...	dee REE-zee-ken zint...
Bleeding	Bluten	BLOOT-en
Infection	Infektion	in-fek-TS-YON
Scar	Narbe	NAR-be
Repeat procedure	Wiederholung des Eingriffs	vee-der-HOL-oong das AYN-grifs
Iodine	Jod	YOD
Damage to your... (See Body Parts List)	Beschädigung des	be-SHEY-dee-goong des
Sign here	Unterschreiben Sie hier	oon-ter-SH-RAY-ben zee heer
TESTS		
X-ray	Röntgenaufnahme	RUNT-gen-AUF-na-me
C.A.T. Scan	Tomografie	TO-mo-gra-FEE
Ultrasound	Ultraschall	OOL-tra-shal
Catheterization/ bladder catheter	Katheterlegung/Blasenkatheter	ka-te-ter-LE-goong / BLA-zen-ka-te-ter

(cont.)

74 German—Deutsch

Colonoscopy (from below)/Endoscopy (from above)	Darmspiegelung	darm-SH-PEE-ge-loong
Endoscopy	Endoskopie	en-do-sko-PEE
END OF LIFE		
Do you want us to…	Möchten Sie das wir…	MUKH-ten zee das veer…
Perform CPR	Wiederbelebungsversuche durchführen	VEE-der-be-LEY-boongs-fer-ZOO-khe door-kh-FÜR-en
Defibrillate	Sie Defibrillieren	zee de-fib-re-LEE-ren
Intubate	Sie intubieren	zee in-too-BEE-ren?
He/she is dead	Er/Sie ist tot	er /zee ist TOT
We did all we could	Wir haben alles gemacht, was wir konnten	veer HA-ben AL-les ge-MAKH-t, das veer KON-ten
DISCHARGE		
You have…(See Medical Prob List)	Sie haben…	zee HA-ben…
He/she is going to stay in the hospital	Er/Sie wird im Krankenhaus bleiben	er/zee vird im KRAN-ken-HAUS BLAY-ben
Take "X" pills "Y" times a day for "Z" days	Nehmen Sie "X" Pillen "Y" Mal pro Tag für "Z" Tage	NEY-men zee "X" PIL-len "Y" mal pro tak für "Z" TA-ge
Pills	Pillen / Tabletten	PIL-len / tab-LEYT-ten
Antibiotics	Antibiotika	AN-tee-BEE-O-tee-ka
Before/after meals	Vor/nach Mahlzeiten	for/nakh MAL-tsay-ten
Return to the ER if…	Kehren Sie zum Notarzt zurück, wenn	KE-ren zee zum NOT-ahrtst tsoo-RÜK, ven
Follow up at "X" on "Y"	Machen Sie einen Folgetermin bei "X" am "Y"	MA-khen zee AYN-en fol-ge-TER-meen bay "X" am "Y"
You're welcome	Keine Ursache	KAY-ne OOR-za-khe

German—Deutsch

Goodbye	Auf Wiedersehen	auf VEE-der-ZAY-en
MEDICAL PROBS		
AIDS/HIV	AIDS/HIV	eydz (a-ee-dey-es) / ha-ee-fau
Anemia	Anämie	a-NEY-mee-e
Arrhythmia	Herzrhythmusstörung	her-ts-rit-moos-sh-TER-oonk
Arthritis	Arthritis	ar-TREE-tis
Asthma	Asthma	AST-ma
Bronchitis	Bronchitis	bron-KEE-tis
Cancer	Krebs	kreyp-s
Cirrosis	Zirrhose	TSEER-ro-se
Cholesterol	Cholesterin	KO-les-ter-EEN
Cold	Erkältung	AYR-kelt-oong
Constipation	Verstopfung	fer-SH-TOP-foong
Cyst	Zyste	TSIS-te
Diabetes	Diabetes	DEE-a-BEY-tes
Dialysis	Dialyse / Blutwäsche	DEE-a-LÜ-se / BLOOT-vesh-e
Diverticulitis	Divertikulitis	DEE-ver-TIK-oo-LEE-tis
Emphysema	Emphysem	em-FÜ-seym
Fibroids	Fibriosis / Gebärmuttermyome	FEE-bree-O-sis / ge-BER-moot-ter-moo-o-me
Fracture	Bruch	brukh
Flu	Grippe	GRIP-pe
Gallstones	Gallensteine	GAL-len-SH-TAY-ne
Gastritis/GERD	Gastritis/Refluxösophagitis	gas-TREE-tis/REY-flooks-Ü-so-fa-GEE-tis

(cont.)

Hepatitis	Hepatitis	hep-a-TEE-tis
Heart attack	Herzinfarkt	HERTS-in-farkt
Heart disease	Herzkrankheit	HERTS-krank-hayt
Heart failure	Herzversagen	herts-fer-ZA-gen
Hypertension	Hoher Blutdruck	HO-er BLOOT-drook
Indigestion	Magenverstimmung	MA-gen-fer-SH-TIM-moong
Kidney stone	Nierenstein	NEE-ren-sh-tayn
Lupus	Lupus	LOO-poos
Migraine	Migräne	mee-GRAY-ne
Murmur	Murmel / Auskultationsgeräusch	MOOR-mel / aus-kul-TA-tsee-ONZ-ge-roysh
Pacemaker	Schrittmacher	SH-RIT-makh-er
Pneumonia	Lungenentzündung	LOONG-en-en-TSÜN-doong
Seizures	Ergreifungen / Starrkrämpfe	er-GRAY-foong-en
STD	Sexuell übertragene Krankheit / Geschlechtskrankheit	zek-SOO-el ü-ber-TRA-ge-ne KRANK-hayt / gesh-LEKH-ts-krank-hayt
Stroke	Schlaganfall	SH-LAG-an-fal
Ulcer	Geschwür	ge-SH-VÜR
Ulcerative colitis	Colitis ulcerosa	KOL-ee-tis OOL-ser-O-sa
UTI	Harnwegsinfektion	harn-vegs-IN-FEK-ts-yoon
BODY PARTS		
Abdomen	Bauch	baukh
Ankle	Knöchel	K-NU-khel
Appendix	Blinddarm	blint-darm
Arm	Arm	arm

Artery	Ader / Arterie	ader / ahr-TER-ee-eh
Back	Rücken	RÜK-en
Bladder	Blase	BLA-ze
Blood	Blut	BLOOT
Bone	Knochen	K-NOKH-en
Brain	Gehirn	ge-HIRN
Breast	Brust	broost
Calf	Wade	VA-de
Chest	Brustkorb	BROOST-korb
Chin	Kinn	kin
Ear	Ohr	or
Elbow	Ellenbogen	EL-len-BO-gen
Eye	Auge	AU-ge
Face	Gesicht	ge-ZIKH-T
Finger	Finger	FING-er
Foot	Fuss	foos
Hand	Hand	hant
Head	Kopf	kop-f
Heart	Hertz	herts
Gallbladder	Gallenblase	GAL-len-BLA-ze
Jaw	Kiefer	KEE-fer
Joint	Gelenk	ge-LENK
Kidney	Niere	NEE-re
Knee	Knie	k-nee
Leg	Bein	bayn
Liver	Leber	LEY-ber

(cont.)

Mouth	Mund	moont
Muscle	Muskel	MOOS-kel
Neck	Nacken	NAK-ken
Nerve	Nerv	nerv
Nose	Nase	NA-se
Ovary	Eierstock	AY-er-sh-tok
Pancreas	Bauchspeicheldrüse	BAUKH-sh-pay-khel-DRÜ-ze
Penis	Penis	PEY-nis
Prostate	Prostata	PROS-ta-ta
Rectum	Mastdarm	MAST-darm
Rib	Rippe	RIP-pe
Shoulder	Schulter	SHOOL-ter
Skin	Haut	haut
Spleen	Milz	mil-ts
Spine	Wirbelsäule	VIR-bel-ZOY-le
Stomach	Magen	MA-gen
Teeth	Zähne	tsey-ne
Testicle	Hoden	HO-den
Throat	Kehle	KEY-le
Thyroid	Schilddrüse	SHILD-drü-ze
Toe	Zeh	tse
Tonsils	Mandeln	MAN-deln
Tongue	Zunge	TSOON-ge
Uterus	Gebärmutter	ge-BER-moo-ter
Vagina	Scheide	SHAY-de
Vein	Vene	VEY-ne

Wrist	Handgelenk	hant-ge-LENK

NUMBERS

How many (times)?	Wie viel Mal?	vee feel mal?
0	Null	nool
1	Ein	ayn
2	Zwei	tsvay
3	Drei	dray
4	Vier	feer
5	Fünf	fünf
6	Sechs	zek-s
7	Sieben	ZEE-ben
8	Acht	akh-t
9	Neun	noyn
10	Zehn	tseyn
11	Elf	elf
20	Zwanzig	TZ-VAN-tseek
30	Dreizig	DRAY-tseek
40	Vierzig	FEER-tseek
50	Fünfzig	FÜNF-tseek
60	Sechzig	ZEK-tseek
70	Siebzig	ZEEP-tseek
80	Achtzig	AKH-tseek
90	Neunzig	NOYN-tseek
100	Ein Hundert	ayn HOON-dert

Hindi — हिंदी

WORD/PHRASE	TRANSLATION	ENGLISH PRONUNCIATION
Hindi	हिन्दी	hin-dee
INTRODUCTION & REGISTRATION		
Hello	नमस्ते	na-ma-STE
I am doctor/nurse (add your name)	मै डाक्टर / नर्स _____ हूँ	MAYN dok-tor (doctor) / ners (nurse) (add your name) hoon
What is your name?	आपका नाम क्या हैं	op-KA nam k-ya HAY
Who is your doctor?	आपका डाक्टर कौन हैं	op-KA dok-tor kon HAY
How old are you?	आपकी उमर कितनी हैं	op-KEE oo-mar kit-NEE HAY
Birthdate?	जन्मदिन	jan-NAM din
Telephone number?	टैलिफोन नम्बर	te-le-FON NUM-ber
Address?	पता	pa-TA
Social security number?	कार्ड नम्बर	kard NUM-ber
Insurance?	बीमा	bee-MA
BASICS		
Do you understand?	क्या आपको समझ में आया	k-ya op-KO sa-muj MEY a-YA
Yes	हाँ	ha
No	नहीं	NA-hee
Please	कृपया	krip-YA
Thank you	धन्यवाद्	DUN-ya vad

(cont.)

Sorry	माफी	MA-fee
I don't understand	मुझे समझ में नहीं आया	moo-JE sa-muj MAYN na-HEEN a-YA
Repeat	फिर से कहना	feer-SAY ke-NA
Speak slowly	धीरे बोलो	deer-E bo-LO
Answer "yes" or "no"	बोलो हाँ या ना	bo-LO ha YA NA
Here	यहाँ	ya-ha
This	यह	YEY
It's alright (consoling)	कोई नहीं	ko-EE na-HEE
I'll be right back	मै वापस जलदी आऊगी	MAY va-pus jul-DEE aj-a-GEE

GENERAL

What's wrong?	क्या मुसकिल हैं	k-ya mus-kil HAY
Pain	दर्द	da-UR-da
Do you have pain?	क्या आपको दर्द हैं	k-ya op-KO da-UR-da HAY
Does the pain radiate?	क्या दर्द हिलती हैं	k-ya da-UR-da hil-tee HAY
Where (show me)	दिखाओ किधर हैं	dik-AW ki-DER hay
Gone now	अब चली गई	ub cha-LEE ga-EE
Still present	अभी हैं	ub-EE HAY
Sudden/gradual onset	अचानक / धीरे–धीरे	A-chan-nuk / dee-RE-dee-RE
What bothers you the most?	आपको सबसे ज्याढा क्या फिकर हैं	op-KO sub-SE za-DA k-ya fee-kur HAY
Why did you come today?	आप आज क्यो आए हो	op A-ju kyoo A-ya ho

Hindi — हिंदी

QUALITY		
If '0' is no pain and 10 is maximum pain, what number do you have now?	अगर शून्य कम दर्द है और दस सबस ज्यादा दर्द है, अभी आपका दर्द कितना है	u-gur shun-YA kum da-UR-da HAY or dus zya-da da-UR-da HAY, u-bhee op-KA da-UR-da kit-NA HAY
Burning	जलन	JA-lan
Constant	लगातार	la-GA-tar
Dull	सुस्त	soos-TA
Intermittent	कभी—कभी	ka-BEE-ka-BEE
Pressure	ढबाव	DU-bav
Severe	गंभीर	gum-BEER
Sharp/prickly	तेज / कंटीला	te-ZE / KUM-tee-LA
Throbbing	टीस	teez
ASSOCIATED SYMPTOMS		
Onset during... (before/after)	पहले / बाद...	pe-LE / bad...
Worse (with...)	बेहतर (...के साथ)	BUD-tur ... KAY saat
Better (with...)	बेहतर (...के साथ)	BEY-tur ... KAY saat
Cough	खाँसी	ka-SEE
Deep breath	लंबा साँस	lum-ba san-sa
Emotional upset	भावुक परेशानी	ba-VOOK par-E-sha-NEE
Food	खाना	ka-NA
Movement	हरकत	hur-kut

(cont.)

Nothing	कुछ नहीं	kooch na-HEE
Positioning	दिशा	DI-sha
Rest	आराम	A-ram-a
Walking	चलना	chul-NA

TIME COURSE

For how long?	कितनी देर	kit-NEE der
Today	आज	A-ja
Yesterday	कल	kul
How many...	कितनी...	kit-NEE...
Months/weeks/days/hours/seconds	महीना / हफ्ता / दिन / घंटा / सेकंड	ma-HEE-na/huf-ta/din/gan-TA/SE-kund
Still present?	अभी हैं	ub-EE HAY
Gone now?	चली गई	cha-LEE ga-EE
How long did it last? (see Numbers)	कितनी देर रही	kit-NEE der ra-HEE
Have you had this before?	पहले भी था	pe-LE BEE TA
How many times?	कितनी बार	kit-NEE bar
When was the last time?	आखरी समह	AK-ree sum-E
New	नया	na-YA
Old	पुराना	poo-RA-na

CONTEXT

Did you...?	क्या आप...	k-ya op...
fall	गिरे	gir-E
trip	फिसले	fis-LE

Hindi — हिंदी

faint	बेहोश	be-hosh
twist	बल खाया	bul ka-YA
get hit	को मारा	ko ma-RA
get burned	जले	ja-LE
get assaulted	हमला हुआ	hum-LA hoo-A
get bitten	काटा	ka-TA
PAST MEDICAL HISTORY		
Take medication?	क्या आप कोई दवा ले रहे हैं	k-ya op koy da-wa LE ra-HE HAYN
(aspirin/antibiotics)	(एस्प्रीन / एंटिबायोटिक)	(as-per-IN/an-ti-bay-O-tik)
Do you have... (see Medical Problems)	क्या आपको_____हैं	k-ya op-ko ___ HAY
allergies	एलर्जी	el-ER-zee
medical problems	बीमारी	BEE-mar-ee
Do you have problems of the ... (see Body Parts)	क्या आपको____की बीमारी हैं	kya op-KO ___ KEE BEE-mar-ee HAY
SURGICAL HISTORY		
Have you had surgery?	क्या आपकी चीर–फार हुई हैं	k-ya op-KEE CHEER far hoo-EE HAY
Surgery on...(see Body Parts)	_____चीर–फार हुई हैं	___ pey CHEER far hoo-EE HAY
SOCIAL HISTORY		
Smoke?	सिग्रेट	sig-rut?
Drink?	शराब पीना	sh-rab pee-NA?
Take drugs?	नशीली दवा लेना	na-see-lee da-wa LE-na?

(cont.)

Recent travel?	हाल का यात्रा	hal ka YA-tra?
Are you sexually active?	क्या आप संभोग करते हो	k-ya op sam-bog kur-TE ho?
Do you use condoms?	क्या आप निरोध इस्तेमाल करते हो	k-ya op NIR-od is-TE-mal kur-TE ho?
Homosexual	समलिंगी	sum-ling-EE

SYSTEMS REVIEW

Do you have...	क्या आपको____हैं	k-ya op-ko __ HAY

GENERAL

Fever	बुखार	BOO-kar
Chills	थंड	ta-UND
Weight loss	वज़न कम	vaz-UN kum
Fatigue	थकवाट	ta-KA-vut
Sick contact	बीमार मिला हैं	BEE-mar mee-LA HAY

HEENT

Sore throat	गले में दर्द	gu-LE MEYN da-ER-da
Runny nose	नाक बहना	nuk be-NA
Nosebleed	नाक से खून	nuk SE koon
Ear pain	कान में दर्द	ka-NA MEYN da-UR-da
Ear ringing	कान में आवाज़	ka-NA MEYN A-waz
Decreased hearing	कम सुनना	kum soon-NA

EYE

Eye pain	आँख में दर्द	AUK MEYN da-UR-da
Blurry vision	धुंधला दीखना	doon-d-LA deek-NA

Hindi — हिंदी

Diplopia	दुगुना दीखना	doog-NA deek-NA
Foreign body sensation	आपको कुच अजीब लग रहा हैं	op-KO kooch U-jeeb lug ru-ha HAY
Contact lenses	कोंटेकत लेनस	kan-tact lens
CARDIAC		
Chest pain	छाती में दर्द	cha-TEE MEYN da-UR-da
Palpitations	तेज धड़कन	taj durk-EN
Orthopnea	लेटके सांस कम होन	LET-KE kum san-sa ho-NA
Dyspnea on exertion	काम करते सांस कम होन	kam kur-TE san-sa kum ho-NA
Fainting (syncope)	बेहोश हो जाना	be-hosh ho ja-NA
Leg swelling	टाँग में सुजन	tong MEYN soo-JUN
How many pillows?	कितने तकिय	kit-NEE ta-KEE-YA?
PULMONARY		
Trouble breathing	सांस में मुश्किल	san-sa MEYN mus-kil
SOB	कम सांस लेना	kum san-sa LAY-na
Cough	खाँसी	ka-SEE
Sputum	थूक	TOOK-ka
Pain on inspiration	सांस लेते दर्द होन	san-sa le-TEY da-UR-da ho-NA
Hemoptysis	खाँसी में खून	ka-SEE MEYN koon
GI		
Abdominal pain	पेट में दर्द	pet MEYN da-UR-da
Nausea	जी कच्चा होन	jee ka-cha ho-NA

(cont.)

Vomiting	उलटी	ool-TEE
Vomiting blood	उलटी में खून	ool-TEE MEYN koon
Coffee ground emesis	कॉफी जैसी उलटी	kaw-fee ja-SEE ool-TEE
Anorexia	अक्षुधा	a-SOO-dra
Diarrhea	दस्त	dust
Difficulty swallowing	नगलने में मुझिकल	nee-gal-NE MEYN mus-kil
BRBPR	पखाने में लाल खून	fa-ka-NA MEYN lol koon
Melena	गहरा पखान	ga-RA fa-ka-NA
Pain after eating	खाना के बाढ दर्द	ka-NA ke bad da-UR-da
Worms	कीरा	kee-RA
Constipation	कब्ज़	ka-buz

GU

Painful urination	पेशाब करते दर्द	pe-SHAB kur-TE da-UR-da
Urgent urination	पेशाब तेज आना	pe-SHAB tej au-NA
Frequent urination	बार-बार पेशाब करना	bar-bar pe-SHAB kur-NA
Bloody urination	पेशाब में खून	pe-SHAB MEYN koon
Discharge: vaginal/penile	पदात	pa-DA-rut

PSYCH

Anxiety	चन्ता	chin-TA
Depression	उदासी	oo-DA-see
Suicidal thoughts	आत्महत्या करने का विचार	AT-ma-hut-ya kur-NE ka vee-char
Homicidal thoughts	कत्ल करने का विचार	kat-ul kur-NE ka vee-char
Medication overdose	दवा का अधिक लेना	da-wa ka A-deek LE-na

Hindi — हिन्दी

Hear voices	आवाजे सुनना	A-vaz sun-NA
NEURO		
Headache	सिर दर्द	sir da-UR-da
Worst headache of life	सबसे बुरा सिर दर्द	sub-SE bu-RA sir da-UR-da
Weakness	कमजोरी	kum-zor-EE
Dizzy	चक्कर आना	cha-kar aw-NA
What is your name?	आपका नाम क्या हैं	op-KA nam k-ya HAY
Where are we?	हम कहाँ हैं	hum ka-HA HAY
What is the year/month/date?	क्या साल / महीना / दिन हैं	k-ya sa l / ma-HEE-na / din HAY
Bowel dysfunction	पखाने में मुश्किल	fa-ka-NE MEYN mus-kil
Bladder dysfunction	पेशाब में मुश्किल	pe-SHAB MEYN mus-kil
Photophobia	रोशने शे परेशानी	ro-sha-NEE SE pur-ee-saw-NEE
Tingling/numbness	नमनस	NUM-nus
Decreased strength in...(See Body Part List)	शाक्ति का कम होना...में	shuk-TEE ka kum ho-NA ... MEYN
Seizure	मरगी का दौरा	mi-ri-GE ka du-o-ra
Difficulty walking	पैदल चलने में मुश्किल	pe-DAL CHAL-nee MEYN mus-kil
Difficulty speaking	बात करने में मुश्किल	bat KUR-ne MEYN mus-kil
Spinning (vertigo)	चक्कर	chuk-ER
Confusion	दूविधा में पड जाना	DOO-VEE-da MEYN pud ja-na
MISC		
Lump	समूह	su-MU-hu

(cont.)

Itching	खुजली	kuj-lee
Bruising	घाव	gav
Rash	चकता	chu-ka-TA
Swelling	सुजन	soo-JUN
Jaundice	पीलिया	pee-lee-YA

GYNECOLOGIC

Vaginal bleeding	योनि से खून निकलना	yo-NEE SEY koon nee-kul-NA
Heavy	भारी	ba-REE
Irregular	कभी—कभी	ka-BEE-ka-BEE
Absent	गैरहाज़िर	ger-HA-zir
Vaginal discharge	योनि से पदार्त निकलना	yo-NEE SE pa-DA-rut nee-kul-NA
Pelvic pain	माहवारी का दर्द	ma-wa-REE MEY da-UR-da
Rape	बलात्कार	ba-lit-kar
Pain with intercourse	संभोग करते दर्द	kur-TEY da-UR-da
Contraceptive	गर्भ निरोधक	ger-b nee-RO-duk

OBSTETRIC

Are you pregnant?	क्या आप गर्भवती हैं	k-ya op gerb-va-TEE HAY?
LMP how many days ago?	कितनी दिन पहले माहवारी हुई	kit-NEE din pey-LE ma-wa-REE hoo-EE?
Times pregnant?	कितनी बार गर्भवती	kit-NEE bar ger-b-va-TEE?
Times delivered?	कितनी बार बच्चे	kit-NEE bar ba-che?
Miscarriage	गर्भपात	gur-bha-PUT

Abortion	बच्चा गिराया	ba-cha gee-RA-YA
Fluid leakage	तरल निकलना	ta-RA-LU nee-kul-NA
Contraction	संकुचन	sun-koo-CHUN
Fetal movement	बच्चा हिलना	ba-cha hil-NA

TRAUMA

How many hours ago did you eat last?	कितनी घंटा पहले खया	kit-NEE gan-TA pey-LEY ka-YA?
Lost consciousness?	चतना खोना	chut-NA ko-NA?
Tetanus within 5 years?	टेटनस 5 साल के बीच	TET-nus pan-che sal KEY beech?

PEDIATRIC

How old?	कितनी उमर हैं	kit-NEE oo-mar HEY?
Vaccines up to date?	टीका अद्यतन	tee-KA ad-ya-ta-NA?
Urinating normally	पेशाब ठीक हैं	pe-sab teek HEY
Taking liquids	तरल पदार्थ लो	ta-RA-LA pa-DAR-t loo
Increased crying	अधिक रोना	a-dee-ka ro-NA
Ingestion	खाना	KA-na
Foreign body	बाहर की चीज़	buh-har KEE chee-se
Premature	समय से पहले	sum-EY se pe-LE
Birth complications	जन्म के समय उलजन	jan-MAH ke sum-E ool-ja-NE

PHYSICAL EXAM/INSTRUCTION

Sit down (please)	आप बैठिए	op bat-YE

(cont.)

Lie down	लेट जाओ	LET ja-oo
Come here	यहँ आओ	ya-ha a-O
Relax	आराम	a-ram-a
Don't move	हिलो मत	hil-O mut
Open your mouth	अपना मुँह खोलो	up-NA moo ko-LO
Say "ahh"	बोलो "अह्ह"	bo-lo "ahh"
Swallow	निगलो	nig-LO
Breath deeply	गहरी साँस लो	ge-ri san-sa LO
Hold your breath	साँस को रोको	san-sa ko RO-ko
Cough	खाँसी	ka-SEE
Push	धकेलो	da-ke-LO
Pull	खींचो	KEE-cho
Follow my finger	मेरी उगली की तरफ देखो	me-REE oon-GLEE kee ta-RUF de-KO
Close your eyes	अपनी आँखे बन्द करो	up-NEE a-ke bund ka-RO
Smile	मुस्कराओ	mus-ka-RA-o
Can you feel this?	क्या महसूस होता हैं	k-ya me-soos ho-TA HAY?
Copy this (movement)	नकल करो	nuk-ul ka-RO
I am going to put a finger in your rectum	मैं आपका गुदा-सम्बन्धी में उंगली दलने वाला हूँ	MAYN op-KA goo-DA sa-band-EE MAYN oon-GLEE da-lu-ney wa-la hu
I am going to examine your vagina	मैं आपकी योनी की जांच करने वाला ह	MAYN op-KEE yo-NEE KEE ja-ch kur-ney wa-la hu
REASSESSMENT		
Do you feel better?	क्या आपको बेहतर लगत हैं	k-ya op-KO BEY-tur lug-TA HAY?

Do you feel worse?	क्या आपको बढतर लगत हैं	k-ya op-KO BUD-tur lug-TA HAY?
PATIENT WORDS		
I hurt	मुझे चोट लगी हैं	moo-je CHO-ta la-gee HAY
Help!	मढढ	ma-dud!
Bathroom	गुसलखाना	gu-sal-ka-NA
Food	खाना	ka-NA
Water	पानी	pa-NEE
PROCEDURES & CONSENT		
You need...	आपको ज़रूरत हैं.....की	op-KO za-RU-rat HAY... KEE
Injection	टीका	tee-KA
Stiches	टीनके	tin-KE
Cast	पलस्तर	plus-tar
Crutches	बशाखी	BA-sha-kee
Perform surgery on (See Body Parts)	चीर–फार कुरने हैं....पर	CHEER far kur-NEE HAY... pur
The risks are...	खतरे हैं...	kut-RE HAY...
Bleeding	खून बेहना	koon be-NA
Infection	संक्रमण	sun-KRA-man
Scar	निशान	nee-SHAN
Repeat procedure	विधी दोबारा करना	vi-DEE doo-ba-ra kar-na
Iodine	आयोडिन	ay-u-DAYN

(cont.)

Damage to (see Body Parts)	नुकसान होना	nukh-san ho-na
Sign here	हस्ताच्चर करो	hus-ta-kar ka-RO

TESTS

X-ray	एक्सरे	x-ray
C.A.T. Scan	सीटी स्कैन	C.T. scan
Ultrasound	पराध्वनि	per-AD-va-nee
Catheterization/bladder catheter	मूत्राशय का कैथेटर	mut-RA-sha-ya ka kæ-te-tur
Colonoscopy	आँत की जांच	ant KEE ja-ch
Endoscopy	एंडोस्कोपी	en-do-sko-PEE

END OF LIFE

Do you want us to…	क्या आप…करवाना चाहते हो	k-ya op … kur-va-NA cha-TE ho
Perform CPR	CPR करना	see-pee-ER KUR-a-na
Defibrillate	दीफीबरीलेट	de-fib-ril-leyt
Intubate	नली लगाना	nu-lee lu-ga-na
He/she is dead	वह मर गया	vo mur GA-ya
We did all we could	हमने पुरी कोशिश की	hum-NE poo-REE KO-shish KEE

DISCHARGE

You have…(See Medical Prob List)	आपको…हैं	op-KO…HAY
He/she is going to stay in the hospital	मारीज को हस्पताल में रूकना परेगा	ma-ree-ja ko A-pi-tal me rook-NA pur-e-ga
Take "X" pills "Y" times a day for "Z" days	"X" गोली लें "Y" बार दिन में "Z" दिन के लिए	"X" go-lee lay "Y" bar din MEY "Z" din kay lee-yay

Pills	गोली	go-lee
Antibiotics	एंटिबायोटिक	an-ti-bay-ot-ik
Before/after meals	खाना के पहले / बाढ	ka-NA ke pe-LE / bad
Return to the ER if...	ER में वापस आना अगर...	ER MEYN VA-pus a-na u-gur...
Follow up at "X" on "Y"	दोबारा आना "Y" (time) पे, "Y" (day) पे	doo-ba-ra a-na "Y" (time) pey, or "Y" (day) pey "X"
You're welcome	आपक स्वागत हैं	op-KA swa-gut HAY
Goodbye	नमस्ते	na-ma-STE

MEDICAL PROBS

AIDS/HIV	एड्स का रोग	eyd-z ka ro-ga
Anemia	अरक्तता	ar-uk-ta-TA
Arrhythmia	ढिल में अजीब सी धड़कन	dil MEYN U-jeeb see dud-kun
Arthritis	गठिया	GA-tee-ya
Asthma	ढमा	dum
Bronchitis	फेफडे की सूजन	fe-fa-re KEE soo-JUN
Cancer	कैंसर	KAN-sir
Cirrhosis	सूत्रण रोग	soo-tra-na ro-ga
Cholesterol	कोलेस्टेरोल	kol-es-ter-AL
Cold	सर्दी	SUR-dee
Constipation	कब्ज़	KA-buz
Cyst	पीप की थैली	peep KEE TA-lee
Diabetes	मधुमेह	ma-du-me

Hindi — हिंदी

Dialysis	खून की सफाई	koon KEE su-fa-yee
Diverticulitis	एक तरह का आँत की संक्रमण	eyk tu-rah KA ant KEE sun-KRA-man
Emphysema	एम्फ्सीमा	em-fee-see-ma
Fibroids	बच्चेदानी में गाँठ	bu-che-da-NEE MEYN gat
Fracture	टुटना	tut-NA
Flu	फ़्लू	floo
Gallstones	पित्ताशय के पत्थर	pit-TAS-ya kay put-TAR
Gastritis/GERD	गैस्ट्राडटिस	gas-TREE-tees
Hepatitis	कलेजे की सूजन	ku-ley-jey KEE soo-JUN
Heart attack	दिल का दौरा	dil ka dau-RA
Heart disease	दिल की बीमारी	dil KEE BEE-mar-EE
Heart failure	दिल का काम न करना	dil ka kam na kur-NA
Hypertension	रक्तचाप	rak-chup
Indigestion	बदहज़मी	bud-huz-me
Kidney stone	गुर्दे क पत्थर	gur-DA ka put-TAR
Lupus	लूपस	loo-pus
Migraine	माइग्रेन	may-gren
Murmur	दिल में अजीब सी आवाज़	dil MEYN U-jeeb see A-WA-z
Pacemaker	गति नियामक	ga-tee nee-YA-ma-ka
Pneumonia	निमोनिया	noo-mo-NEE-YA
Seizures	दौरा	do-RA

STD	जातीय रोग	ja-TEE-yu ro-ga
Stroke	अधरंग	ud-run-gu
Ulcer	नासूर	na-sur
Ulcerative colitis	आँत में सुजन	ant MEYN soo-JUN
UTI	मूत्रपथ में संक्रमण (यूटीआई)	moo-tru-put MAYN sun-KRA-man (UTI)
BODY PARTS		
Abdomen	पेट	pet
Ankle	टखना	tuk-NA
Appendix	अपेंडिक्स	u-pen-diks
Arm	बाँह	ba
Artery	धमनी	dum-NEE
Back	पीठ	pe-te
Bladder	मूत्राशय	mut-RA-sha-ya
Blood	खून	koon
Bone	हड्डी	hud-DEE
Brain	ढिमाग	DEE-mag
Breast	स्तन	sa-tun
Calf	पिंडली	pin-da-lee
Chest	सीना	see-NA
Chin	ठोडी	to-DEE
Ear	कान	kan

(cont.)

Elbow	कुहनी	ku-NEE
Eye	आंख	ANK
Face	चेहरा	che-RA
Finger	उंगली	oon-GLEE
Foot	पैर	per
Hand	हाथ	ha-ta
Head	सिर	sir
Heart	ढिल	dil
Gallbladder	पित्ताशय	pit-TAS-ya
Jaw	जबडा	ju-BA-da
Joint	जोड	jo-de
Kidney	गुर्ढ	gur-DA
Knee	घुटना	goot-NA
Leg	पैर	per
Liver	कलेजा	ka-le-JA
Mouth	मुँह	moon
Muscle	माँसपेषी	man-sa-pe-SHEE
Neck	गर्ढन	gur-den
Nerve	नस	nus
Nose	नाक	nak
Ovary	अन्डाशय	un-DA-sha

Pancreas	पेट में पाचन–रस की थैली	pet MEY pa-chun-rus KEE ta-lee
Penis	लिंग	ling
Prostate	पुरस्थ ग्रंथि	pur-US-ta GRAN-tee
Rectum	गुदा–सम्बन्धी	goo-DA sa-band-EE
Rib	पसली	PUS-lee
Shoulder	कंधा	KAN-du
Skin	चमड़ी	chum-DEE
Spleen	पलीहा	pa-lee-HA
Spine	रीढ़ की हड्डी	reed KEE hud-DEE
Stomach	पेट	pet
Teeth	दाँत	dant
Testicle	अण्डकोष	und-kosh
Throat	गला	ga-la
Thyroid	गला ग्रंथि	ga-la gran-TEE
Toe	पंजा	pun-ja
Tonsils	टांसिल	ton-sul
Tongue	जीभ	jee-bu
Uterus	बच्चेदानी	bu-che-da-NEE
Vagina	योनी	yo-NEE
Vein	नस	nus
Wrist	कलाई	ka-lay

(cont.)

Hindi — हिंदी

NUMBERS		
How many (times)?	कितने हैं	kit-NEE HAY
0	शून्य	shun-YA
1	एक	eyk
2	दो	do
3	तीन	teen
4	चार	char
5	पाँच	pan-che
6	छह्	che
7	सात	sat
8	आट	aw-t
9	नौ	no
10	दस	dus
11	गयारह	ga-ya-RA
20	बीस	bees
30	तीस	tees
40	चालीस	cha-lees
50	पचास	pa-chas
60	साट	sa-tu
70	सतर	sut-tur
80	अस्सी	us-see
90	नब्बे	nub-be
100	सौ	sau

Italian—Italiano

WORD/PHRASE	TRANSLATION	ENGLISH PRONUNCIATION
Italian	Italiano	ee-ta-L-YA-no
INTRODUCTION & REGISTRATION		
Hello	Ciao	CHA-o
I am a doctor / nurse *(add your name)*	Sono il dottor / infermier *(add your name)*	SO-no eel dot-TOR / een-fer-M-YER *(add your name)*
What is your name?	Come si chiama?	KO-me see K-YA-ma?
Who is your doctor?	Chi è il suo medico curante?	kee E eel SOO-o ME-dee-ko koo-RAN-te
How old are you?	Quanti anni ha?	KWAN-tee AN-nee a?
Birthdate?	Data di nascita?	DA-ta dee NA-shee-ta?
Telephone number?	Numero di telefono?	NOO-me-ro dee te-LE-fono?
Address?	Indirizzo?	een-dee-REET-tso?
Social security number?	Codice fiscale?	KO-dee-che fee-SKA-le?
Insurance?	Assicurazione?	as-see-koo-ra-TS-YO-ne?
BASICS		
Do you understand?	Capisce quello che dico?	ka-PEE-she KWEL-lo ke DEE-ko?
Yes	Sì	see
No	No	no
Please	Per favore	per fa-VO-re
Thank you	Grazie	GRA-ts-ye
Sorry	Scusi	SKOO-zee
I don't understand	Non capisco	non ka-PEE-sko

(cont.)

Repeat	Ripeta	ree-PE-ta
Speak slowly	Parli piano	PAR-lee P-YA-no
Answer "yes" or "no"	Risponda "sì" o "no"	ree-SPON-da "see" o "no"
Here	Ecco	EK-ko
This	Questo	KWE-sto
It's alright (consoling)	Va bene	va BE-ne
I'll be right back	Torno subito	TOR-no SOO-bee-to

GENERAL

What's wrong?	Che c'è che non va?	ke CHE ke non va?
Pain	Dolore	do-LO-re
Do you have pain?	Le fa male?	le fa MA-le?
Does the pain radiate?	Il dolore si sposta?	eel do-LO-re see SPO-sta?
Where (show me)	Dove?	DO-ve?
Gone now	È andato via?	E an-DA-to vee-a?
Still present	C'è ancora?	che an-KO-ra?
Sudden/gradual onset	È una fitta o un dolore continuo?	E OO-na FEET-ta o oon do-LO-re kon-TEE-noo-o?
What bothers you the most?	Cosa le dà più fastidio?	KO-za le DA P-YOO fa-STEE-dee-o?
Why did you come today?	Per quale ragione è venuto a consultarmi?	per KWA-le ra-JO-ne E ve-NOO-to a kon-sool-TAR-mee?

QUALITY

If '0' is no pain and 10 is maximum pain, what number do you have now?	Su una scala da zero a dieci (il massimo dolore), quanto le fa male?	soo OO-na SKA-la da TSE-ro a dee-EY-chee (eel MAS-see-mo do-LO-re), KWAN-to le fa MA-le?
Burning	Bruciante	broo-CHAN-te
Constant	Costante	ko-STAN-te

Dull	Sordo	SOR-do
Intermittent	Intermittente	een-ter-meet-TEN-te
Pressure	Pressione	pres-S-YO-ne
Severe	Intenso	een-TEN-so
Sharp/prickly pains	Acuto	a-KOO-to
Throbbing	Pulsante	pool-SAN-te
ASSOCIATED SYMPTOMS		
Onset during... (before/after)	È cominciato... (prima di/dopo di)	E ko-meen-CHA-to... (PREE-ma dee/DO-po dee)
Worse (with...)	Peggio (con...)	PEJ-jo (kon...)
Better (with...)	Meglio (con...)	MEL-yo (kon...)
Cough	Tosse	TOS-se
Deep breath	Respiro profondo	re-SPEE-ro pro-FON-do
Emotional upset	Stress emotivo	stres e-mo-TEE-vo
Food	Cibo	CHEE-bo
Movement	Movimento	mo-vee-MEN-to
Nothing	Niente	N-YEN-te
Positioning	Quando cambia posizione?	KWAN-do KAM-b-ya po-zee-TS-YO-ne?
Rest	Riposo	ree-PO-zo
Walking	Camminare	ka-mee-NA-re
TIME COURSE		
For how long?	Per quanto tempo?	per KWAN-to TEM-po?
Today	Oggi	OJ-jee
Yesterday	Ieri	YE-ree
How many...	Per quanti...	per KWAN-tee...

(cont.)

Months/weeks/days/hours/seconds	Mesi/settimane/giorni/ore/secondi	MEY-zee/set-tee-MA-ne/JOR-nee/O-re/se-KON-dee
Still present?	C'è ancora?	che an-KO-ra?
Gone now?	È andato via?	E an-DA-to vee-a?
How long did it last? (See Numbers List)	Per quanto tempo è durato?	per KWAN-to TEM-po E doo-RA-to?
Have you had this before?	Le è mai successo prima?	le E MAY soo-CHES-so PREE-ma?
How many times?	Quante volte?	KWAN-te VOL-te?
When was the last time?	Quando è stata l'ultima volta?	KWAN-do E STA-ta LOOL-tee-ma VOL-ta?
New	Nuovo	noo-O-vo
Old	Vecchio	VEK-kee-o
CONTEXT		
Did you...?	È...?	E...?
fall	È caduto?	E ka-DOO-to?
trip	È inciampato?	E een-cham-PA-to?
faint	È svenuto?	E s-ve-NOO-to?
twist	Ha preso una storta?	A PRE-zo OO-na STOR-ta?
get hit	È stato colpito?	E STA-to col-PEE-to?
get burned	Si è bruciato?	see E broo-CHA-to?
get assaulted	L'hanno aggredita?	LAN-no a-gre-DEE-ta?
get bitten (human/dog/cat/insect)	È stato morso?	E STA-to MOR-so?
PAST MEDICAL HISTORY		
Take medication?	Prende qualche medicina?	PREN-de KWAL-ke me-dee-CHEE-na?
(aspirin/antibiotics)	(aspirina/antibiotici)	as-pee-REE-na/an-tee-bee-O-tee-chee

Do you have (See also Medical Problems List)...	Ha...?	A...?
allergies	allergie	al-ler-JEE-ye
medical problems	problemi di salute	pro-BLE-mee dee sa-LOO-te
Do you have problems of the... (see Body Parts List)	Ha problemi di...	a pro-BLE-mee dee...
SURGICAL HISTORY		
Have you had surgery?	Ha mai subito interventi chirurgici?	A MAY soo-BEE-to eenter-VEN-tee kee-ROOR-jee-chee?
Surgery on/"to remove"...(see Body Parts List)	Operato a...	o-per-A-to a...
SOCIAL HISTORY		
Smoke?	Fuma?	FOO-ma?
Drink?	Beve alcool?	BE-ve al-ko-OL?
Take drugs?	Assume delle droghe?	as-SOO-me DEL-le DRO-ge?
Recent travel?	Ha viaggiato di recente?	a vee-a-JA-to dee re-CHEN-te?
Are you sexually active?	È sessualmente attivo?	E ses-su-al-MEN-te a-TEE-vo?
Do you use condoms?	Usa il preservativo?	OO-za eel pre-ser-va-TEE-vo?
Homosexual	Omosessuale	o-mo-ses-soo-A-le
SYSTEMS REVIEW		
Do you have...	Ha...?	A...?

(cont.)

GENERAL		
Fever	Ha febbre?	A FEB-bre?
Chills	Ha brividi di freddo?	A BREE-vee-dee dee FRED-do?
Weight loss	È dimagrito?	E dee-ma-GREE-to?
Fatigue	Ha stanchezza?	stan-KET-tsa?
Sick contact	È entrato in contatto con altri malati?	E en-TRA-to een kon-TAT-to kon AL-tree ma-LA-tee?
HEENT		
Sore throat	Mal di gola	MAL dee GO-la
Runny nose	Naso che cola	NA-zo ke KO-la
Nosebleed	Sangue dal naso	SAN-g-we dal NA-zo
Ear pain	Dolore alle orecchie	do-LO-re AL-le o-RE-k-ye
Ear ringing	Ronzio alle orecchie	ron-TS-EE-o AL-le o-RE-k-ye
Decreased hearing	Difficoltà uditive	deef-fee-kol-TA oo-dee-TEE-ve
EYE		
Eye pain	Dolore all'occhio	do-LO-re del OK-kee-o
Blurry vision	Vista sfocata	VEE-sta s-fo-KA-ta
Diplopia	Vede doppio?	VE-de DOP-pee-o?
Foreign body sensation	Sente di avere qualcosa nell'occhio?	SEN-te dee a-VE-re kwal-KO-za nell O-k-yo?
Contact lenses	Lenti a contatto	LEN-tee a kon-TAT-to
CARDIAC		
Chest pain	Dolore al petto	do-LO-re al PET-to
Palpitations	Palpitazioni	pal-pee-ta-TS-YO-nee

Orthopnea	Difficoltà a respirare quando si corica	dee-fee-kol-TA a res-pee-RA-re KWAN-do see KO-ree-ka
Dyspnea on exertion	Difficoltà a respirare quando cammina	deef-fee-kol-TA a res-pee-RA-re KWAN-do cam-MEE-na
Fainting (syncope)	Svenimento	s-ve-nee-MEN-to
Leg swelling	Gambe gonfie	GAM-be GON-f-ye
How many pillows?	Con quanti cuscini dorme?	kon KWAN-tee koo-SHEE-nee DOR-me?
PULMONARY		
Trouble breathing	Difficoltà a respirare	deef-fee-kol-TA a re-spee-RA-re
SOB	Le manca il fiato?	le MAN-ka eel fee-A-to?
Cough	Tosse	TOS-se
Sputum	Saliva/Muco	sa-LEE-va/MOO-ko
Pain on inspiration	Dolore quando inspira	do-LO-re KWAN-do een-SPEE-ra
Hemoptysis	Tossisce sangue	to-SEE-she SAN-g-we
GI		
Abdominal pain	Dolori addominali	do-LO-ree ad-do-mee-NA-lee
Nausea	Nausea	NAU-ze-a
Vomiting	Vomito	VO-mee-to
Vomiting blood	Vomita sangue?	VO-mee-ta SAN-g-we?
Coffee ground emesis	Vomito nero e granuloso	VO-mee-to NE-ro e gra-noo-LO-zo
Anorexia	Anoressia	a-no-res-SEE-a
Diarrhea	Diarrea	dee-ar-REY-a

(cont.)

Difficulty swallowing	Difficoltà ad inghiottire	deef-fee-kol-TA ad een-gee-ot-TEE-re
BRBPR	Sangue rosso vivo dal retto	SAN-g-we ROS-so VEE-vo dal RET-to
Melena	Escremento nero che assomiglia al catrame	es-kre-MEN-to NE-ro ke as-so-MEEL-ya al ka-TRA-me
Pain after eating	Dolore dopo aver mangiato	do-LO-re DO-po a-VER man-JA-to
Worms	Vermi	VER-mee
Constipation	Stitichezza	stee-tee-KET-tsa
GU		
Painful urination	Le fa male mentre sta urinando?	le fa MA-le MEN-tre sta oo-ree-NAN-do?
Urgent urination	Deve correre a urinare?	DE-ve KOR-re-re a oo-ree-NA-re?
Frequent urination	Deve urinare spesso?	DE-ve oo-re-NA-re SPES-so?
Bloody urination	Ha del sangue nell'urina?	a del SAN-g-we nel-loo-REE-na?
Discharge: vaginal/penile	Secrezioni vaginali/ dal pene	se-kre-TS-YO-nee va-jee-NA-lee/dal PE-ne
PSYCH		
Anxiety	Angoscia	an-GO-sha
Depression	Depressione	de-pres-S-YO-ne
Suicidal thoughts	Pensa al suicidio	PEN-sa al soo-ee-CHEE-dyo
Homicidal thoughts	Pensa all'omicidio	PEN-sa al-lo-mee-CHEE-dyo
Medication overdose	Overdose	o-ver-DOZ
Hear voices	Sente le voci?	SEN-te le VO-chee?

NEURO		
Headache	Mal di testa	mal dee TES-ta
Worst headache of life	Il peggior mal di testa della vita	eel pe-JOR mal dee TE-sta DEL-la VEE-ta
Weakness	Debolezza	de-bo-LET-tsa
Dizzy	Le gira la testa?	le JEE-ra la TE-sta?
What is your name?	Come si chiama?	KO-me see K-YA-ma?
Where are we?	Dove siamo?	DO-ve S-YA-mo?
What is the year/month/date?	Che anno/mese/giorno è?	ke AN-no/ME-ze/JOR-no E?
Bowel dysfunction	Problemi intestinali	pro-BLE-mee een-te-stee-NA-lee
Bladder dysfunction	Problemi alla vescica	pro-BLE-mee AL-la ve-SHEE-ka
Photophobia	Ha paura della luce?	a pa-U-ra DEL-la LOO-che?
Tingling/numbness	Le si addormentano le gambe/braccia/mani?	le see ad-dor-MEN-ta-no le GAM-be/BRA-cha/MA-nee?
Decreased strength in…(See Body Parts List)	Sente che le si è indebolito il/la/lo…	SEN-te ke le see E een-de-bo-LEE-to eel/la/lo…
Seizure	Convulsioni	kon-vool-SYO-nee
Difficulty walking	Difficoltà a camminare	deef-fee-kol-TA a kam-mee-NA-re
Difficulty speaking	Difficoltà a parlare	deef-fee-kol-TA a par-LA-re
Spinning (vertigo)	Vertigini	ver-TEE-jee-nee
Confusion	Confusione	kon-foo-Z-YO-ne
MISC		
Lump	Nodulo	NO-doo-lo

(cont.)

Itching	Prurito	proo-REE-to
Bruising	Ammaccatura	am-mak-ka-TOO-ra
Rash	Eruzione cutanea	e-roo-TS-YO-ne koo-TA-ne-a
Swelling	Rigonfiamento	ree-gon-f-ya-MEN-to
Jaundice (yellow skin)	Itterizia	eet-te-REE-ts-ya

GYNECOLOGIC

Vaginal bleeding	Perdite di sangue	PER-dee-te dee SAN-g-we
Heavy	Mestruazione pesante	me-stroo-a-TS-YO-ne pe-ZAN-te
Irregular	Mestruazione irregolare	me-stroo-a-TS-YO-ne eer-re-go-LA-re
Absent	Mestruazione assente	me-stroo-a-TS-YO-ne a-SEN-te
Vaginal discharge	Secrezioni vaginali	se-kre-TS-YO-nee va-jee-NA-lee
Pelvic pain	Dolore al bacino	do-LO-re al ba-CHEE-no
Rape	Stupro	STOO-pro
Pain with intercourse	Sente dolore quando fa sesso?	SEN-te do-LO-re KWAN-do fa SES-so
Contraceptive	Contraccettivo	kon-tra-chet-TEE-vo

OBSTETRIC

Are you pregnant?	È incinta?	E een-CHEEN-ta?
LMP how many days ago?	Quanti giorni fa ha avuto le ultime mestruazioni?	KWAN-tee JOR-nee fa a a-VOO-to le OOL-tee-me me-stru-a-TS-YO-nee?
Times pregnant?	Numero di gravidanze?	NOO-me-ro de gra-vee-DAN-tse?
Times delivered?	Quanti parti?	KWAN-tee PAR-tee?
Miscarriage	Aborto spontaneo	a-BOR-to spon-TA-ne-o

Abortion	Aborto (procurato)	a-BOR-to (pro-koo-RA-to)
Fluid leakage	Perdita di liquido?	PER-dee-ta dee LEE-kwee-do
Contraction	Contrazione	kon-tra-TS-YO-ne
Fetal movement	Movimento del feto	mo-vee-MEN-to del FE-to
TRAUMA		
How many hours ago did you eat last?	Quando ha mangiato l'ultima volta?	KWAN-do a man-JA-to LOOL-tee-ma VOL-ta?
Lost consciousness?	Ha perso conoscenza?	a PER-so ko-no-SHEN-tsa?
Tetanus within 5 years?	Tetano negli ultimi cinque anni?	TE-ta-no nel-yee OOL-tee-me CHEEN-kwe AN-nee?
PEDIATRIC		
How old?	Quanti anni ha?	KWAN-tee AN-nee a?
Vaccines up to date?	Quali vaccinazioni ha fatto il bambino?	KWAL-ee va-chee-na-TS-YO-nee a FAT-to eel bam-BEE-no?
Urinating normally	Urina normalmente?	oo-REE-na nor-mal-MEN-te?
Taking liquids	Beve liquidi	BE-ve LEE-kwee-dee
Increased crying	Pianto più frequente	pee-AN-to P-YOO fre-KWEN-te
Ingestion	Ha problemi a ingerire cibi solidi?	a pro-BLE-mee a een-je-REE-re CHEE-bee SO-lee-dee?
Foreign body	Oggetti estranei	o-JET-tee e-STRA-ne-ee
Premature	Prematuro	pre-ma-TOO-ro
Birth complications	Complicazioni del parto	kom-plee-ka-TS-YO-nee del PAR-to

(cont.)

PHYSICAL EXAM/INSTRUCTION		
Sit down (please)	Si sieda (per favore)	see S-YE-da (per fa-VO-re)
Lie down	Si stenda	see STEN-da
Come here	Venga	VEYN-ga
Relax	Si rilassi	see ree-LAS-see
Don't move	Non si muova	non see m-WO-va
Open your mouth	Apra la bocca	A-pra la BOK-ka
Say "ahh"	Dica "aaa"	DEE-ka "aaa"
Swallow	Deglutisca	de-gloo-TEE-ska
Breath deeply	Un respiro profondo	oon re-SPEE-ro pro-FON-do
Hold your breath	Trattenga il respiro	tra-TEYN-ga eel re-SPEE-ro
Cough	Tossisca	tos-SEE-ska
Push	Spinga	SPEEN-ga
Pull	Tiri	TEE-ree
Follow my finger	Segua il dito	SE-g-wa eel DEE-to
Close your eyes	Chiuda gli occhi	kee-OO-da lee OK-kee
Smile	Sorrida	sor-REE-da
Can you feel this?	Lo sente questo?	lo SEN-te KWE-sto?
Copy this (movement)	Faccia questo (movimento)	FA-cha KWE-sto (mo-vee-MEN-to)
I am going to put a finger in your rectum	Devo esaminarle il retto con un dito	DE-vo e-za-mee-NAR-le eel RET-to kon un DEE-to
I am going to examine your vagina	Devo esaminarle la vagina	DE-vo e-za-mee-NAR-le la va-JEE-na
REASSESSMENT		
Do you feel better?	Si sente meglio?	see SEN-te MEL-yo?

Do you feel worse?	Si sente peggio?	see SEN-te PEJ-jo?
PATIENT WORDS		
I hurt	Mi fa male	mee fa MA-le
Help!	Aiuto!	a-YOO-to
Bathroom	Bagno	BAN-yo
Food	Cibo	CHEE-bo
Water	Acqua	A-kwa
PROCEDURES & CONSENT		
You need...	Ha bisogno di...	a bee-ZON-yo dee...
Injection	Iniezione	een-ye-TS-YO-ne
Stiches	Punti di sutura	POON-tee dee soo-TOO-ra
Cast	Gesso	JES-so
Crutches	Stampelle	stam-PEL-le
Perform surgery on the... (See Body Parts List)	Operare a...	o-pe-RA-re a...
The risks are...	I rischi sono...	ee REE-skee SO-no...
Bleeding	Emorragia	e-mor-ra-JEE-a
Infection	Infezione	een-fe-TS-YO-ne
Scar	Cicatrice	chee-ka-TREE-che
Repeat procedure	Ripetere l'operazione	ree-PE-te-re lo-pe-ra-TS-YO-ne
Iodine	Iodio	YO-d-yo
Damage to your... (See Body Parts List)	Danno a _____	DAN-no a _____
Sign here	Firmi qua	FEER-mee kwa
TESTS		
X-ray	raggi X	RAJ-jee eek-ts

(cont.)

C.A.T. Scan	TAC (tomografia assiale computerizzata)	to-mo-gra-FEE-a as-S-YA-le kom-pu-te-ree-TSA-ta
Ultrasound	Ecografia	e-ko-gra-FEE-a
Catheterization/ bladder catheter	Catetere	ka-te-TE-re
Colonoscopy (from below)/Endoscopy (from above)	Colonoscopia	ko-lo-no-sko-PEE-a
Endoscopy	Endoscopia	en-do-sko-PEE-a

END OF LIFE

Do you want us to...	Vuole che ...	V-WO-le ke...
Perform CPR	Rianimare	ree-a-nee-MA-re
Defibrillate	Defibrillare	de-fee-breel-LA-re
Intubate	Intubare	een-too-BA-re
He/she is dead	È morto/a	E MOR-to/ta
We did all we could	Abbiamo fatto tutto il possibile	a-BYA-mo FAT-to TOOT-to eel pos-SEE-bee-le

DISCHARGE

You have...(See Medical Prob List)	Lei ha...	ley a...
He/she is going to stay in the hospital	Lui/lei va a restare in ospedale	loo-ee/ley va a re-STA-re een o-spe-DA-le
Take "X" pills "Y" times a day for "Z" days	Prenda "X" pillole "Y" volte al giorno per "Z" giorni	PREN-da "X" PEEL-lo-le "Y" VOL-te al JOR-no per "Z" JOR-nee
Pills	Pillole	PEEL-lo-le
Antibiotics	Antibiotici	an-tee-bee-O-tee-chee
Before/after meals	Prima/dopo i pasti	PREE-ma/DO-po ee PA-stee

Return to the ER if…	Vada al pronto soccorso se…	VA-da al PRON-to sok-KOR-so se…
Follow up at "X" on "Y"	Torni a "X" il "Y"	TOR-nee a "X" eel "Y"
You're welcome	Prego	PRE-go
Goodbye	Arrivederla	a-ree-ve-DER-la
MEDICAL PROBS		
AIDS/HIV	AIDS/HIV	AY-dz/A-ka ee voo
Anemia	Anemia	a-ne-MEE-a
Arrhythmia	Aritmia	a-reet-MEE-a
Arthritis	Artrite	ar-TREE-te
Asthma	Asma	AZ-ma
Bronchitis	Bronchite	bron-KEE-te
Cancer	Cancro	KAN-kro
Cirrhosis	Cirrosi	cheer-RO-zee
Cholesterol	Colesterolo	ko-le-ste-RO-lo
Cold	Raffreddore	raf-fred-DO-re
Constipation	Stitichezza	stee-tee-KET-tsa
Cyst	Ciste	CHEE-ste
Diabetes	Diabete	d-ya-BE-te
Dialysis	Dialisi	dee-A-lee-zee
Diverticulitis	Diverticolite	dee-ver-tee-ko-LEE-te
Emphysema	Enfisema	en-fee-ZE-ma
Fibroids	Fibroma	fee-BRO-ma
Fracture	Frattura	frat-TOO-ra
Flu	Influenza	een-floo-EN-tsa
Gallstones	Calcoli biliari	KAL-ko-lee bee-L-YA-ree

(cont.)

Gastritis/GERD	Gastrite/Malattia da reflusso gastroesofageo	ga-STREE-te/ma-lat-TEE-a da re-FLOOS-so ga-stro-e-so-fa-JE-o
Hepatitis	Epatite	e-pa-TEE-te
Heart attack	Attacco di cuore	at-TAK-ko dee KWO-re
Heart disease	Malattia di cuore	ma-lat-TEE-a dee KWO-re
Heart failure	Collasso cardiaco	kol-LAS-so kar-DEE-a-ko
Hypertension	Ipertensione	ee-per-ten-S-YO-ne
Indigestion	Indigestione	een-dee-jes-T-YO-ne
Kidney stone	Calcolo renale	KAL-ko-lo re-NA-le
Lupus	Lupus	LOO-poos
Migraine	Emicrania	e-mee-KRA-nee-a
Murmur	Soffio al cuore	SOF-f-yo
Pacemaker	Stimolatore cardiaco	stee-mo-la-TO-re kar-DEE-a-ko
Pneumonia	Polmonite	pol-mo-NEE-te
Seizures	Convulsioni	kon-vool-S-YO-nee
STD	Malattie a trasmissione sessuale	ma-lat-TEE-e a tra-smees-S-YO-ne ses-soo-A-le
Stroke	Ictus	EEK-toos
Ulcer	Ulcera	OOL-che-ra
Ulcerative colitis	Colite ulcerosa	ko-LEE-te ool-che-RO-za
UTI	IAU (infezione dell'apparato urinario)	een-fe-TS-YO-ne del-lap-pa-RA-to oo-ree-NA-ree-o
BODY PARTS		
Abdomen	Addome	ad-DO-me
Ankle	Caviglia	ka-VEEL-ya
Appendix	Appendice	ap-PEN-dee-che

Arm	Braccio	BRA-cho
Artery	Arteria	ar-TE-r-ya
Back	Schiena	SK-YE-na
Bladder	Vescica	ve-SHEE-ka
Blood	Sangue	SAN-g-we
Bone	Osso	OS-so
Brain	Cervello	cher-VEL-lo
Breast	Seno	SE-no
Calf	Polpaccio	pol-PA-cho
Chest	Petto	PET-to
Chin	Mento	MEN-to
Ear	Orecchio	o-RE-k-yo
Elbow	Gomito	GO-mee-to
Eye	Occhio	O-k-yo
Face	Faccia	FA-cha
Finger	Dito	DEE-to
Foot	Piede	P-YE-de
Hand	Mano	MA-no
Head	Testa	TE-sta
Heart	Cuore	KWO-re
Gallbladder	Cistifellea / Colecisti	chee-stee-FEL-le-a / ko-le-CHEE-stee
Jaw	Mascella	ma-SHEL-la
Joint	Articolazione	ar-tee-ko-la-TS-YO-ne
Kidney	Rene	RE-ne
Knee	Ginocchio	jee-NO-k-yo
Leg	Gamba	GAM-ba

(cont.)

Liver	Fegato	FE-ga-to
Mouth	Bocca	BOK-ka
Muscle	Muscolo	MOO-sko-lo
Neck	Collo	KOL-lo
Nerve	Nervo	NER-vo
Nose	Naso	NA-zo
Ovary	Ovaia	o-VAY-a
Pancreas	Pancreas	PAN-kre-as
Penis	Pene	PE-ne
Prostate	Prostata	pro-STRA-ta
Rectum	Retto	RET-to
Rib	Costola	KO-sto-la
Shoulder	Spalla	SPAL-la
Skin	Pelle	PEL-le
Spleen	Milza	MEEL-tsa
Spine	Spina dorsale	SPEE-na dor-SA-le
Stomach	Stomaco	STO-ma-ko
Teeth	Denti	DEN-tee
Testicle	Testicolo	te-STEE-ko-lo
Throat	Gola	GO-la
Thyroid	Tiroide	tee-ROY-de
Toe	Dito del piede	DEE-to del P-YE-de
Tonsils	Tonsille	ton-SEEL-le
Tongue	Lingua	LEEN-gwa
Uterus	Utero	OO-te-ro
Vagina	Vagina	va-JEE-na
Vein	Vena	VE-na

Wrist	Polso	POL-so
NUMBERS		
How many (times)?	Quante (volte)?	KWAN-te (VOL-te)?
0	zero	TSE-ro
1	uno	OO-no
2	due	DOO-e
3	tre	tre
4	quattro	KWAT-tro
5	cinque	CHEEN-kwe
6	sei	sey
7	sette	SET-te
8	otto	OT-to
9	nove	NO-ve
10	dieci	dee-EY-chee
11	undici	OON-dee-chee
20	venti	VAYN-tee
30	trenta	TRAYN-ta
40	quaranta	kwa-RAN-ta
50	cinquanta	cheen-KWAN-ta
60	sessanta	ses-SAN-ta
70	settanta	set-TAN-ta
80	ottanta	ot-TAN-ta
90	novanta	no-VAN-ta
100	cento	CHEN-to

Japanese—日本語

WORD/PHRASE	TRANSLATION	HIRIGANA	ENGLISH PRONUNCIATION
Japanese	日本語		nee-HON-go
INTRODUCTION & REGISTRATION			
Hello	こんにちは		kon-NEE-chee-wa
I am a doctor / nurse	私は担当医師の____です	わたしはたんとういしの____です	wa-TA-shee-wa (EE-sha=doctor)(kan-GO-foo=noor-se) des
What is your name?	お名前は？	おなまえは？	o-NA-ma-e wa nan des-KA?
Who is your doctor?	貴方の主治医は誰ですか？	あなたのしゅじいはだれですか？	a-NA-ta-no shoo-jee-yee-wa DA-re des-KA?
How old are you?	おいくつですか？		oy-KOO-tsoo des-KA?
Birthdate?	生年月日は？	せいねんがっぴは？	SEY-nen-ga-pee-wa EE-tsoo des-KA?
Telephone number?	電話番号を教えてください	でんわばんごうをおしえてください	DEN-wa-ban-go WO O-shee-e-te koo-da-SAY
Address?	住所を教えてください	じゅうしょをおしえてください	joo-sho WO O-shee-e-te koo-da-SAY
Social security number?	ソーシャルセキュリティーナンバーを教えてください		so-sha-roo se-kyoo-ree-tee NAM-ba WO O-shee-e-te koo-da-SAY
Insurance?	保険をお持ちですか？	ほけんをおもちですか？	HO-ken wo o-MO-chee des-KA?
BASICS			
Do you understand?	分かりますか？	わかりますか	wa-ka-ree-mas-ka?
Yes	はい		hay

(cont.)

Japanese—日本語

No	いいえ		ee-E
Please	お願いします	おねがいします	O-ne-gay-shee-mas
Thank you	ありがとうございます		a-ree-GA-TO GO-za-ee-mas
Sorry	すみません		soo-MEE-ma-sen
I don't understand	分かりません	わかりません	wa-ka-REE-ma-sen
Repeat	もう一度お願いします	もういちどおねがいします	mo-ee-CHEE-DO o-NE-ga-ee-shee-mas
Speak slowly	ゆっくり喋って下さい	ゆっくりしゃべってください	YOO-koo-ree SHA-bet-koo-da-sa-ee
Answer "yes" or "no"	「はい」か「いいえ」でお答えください	＿＿＿でおこたえください	"hay" de "ee-E" oko-ta-E-koo-da-sa-ee
Here	ここ		ko-ko
This	これ		ko-re
It's alright (consoling)	大丈夫です	だいじょうぶです	da-ee-JO-boo-des
I'll be right back	すぐ戻ります	すぐもどります	soo-goo-mo-DO-ree-mas

GENERAL

What's wrong?	何処が悪いんですか？	どこがわるいんですか	do-KO-ga-wa-roo-ee-no-des-ka?
Pain	痛み	いたみ	ee-ta-mee?
Do you have pain?	何処か痛みますか？	どこかいたみますか	do-ko-ka-ee-TA-MEE-mas-ka?
Does the pain radiate?	どれぐらいの範囲で痛みますか？	どれぐらいのはんいでいたみますか	do-re-goo-ra-ee-no han-ee-de ee-ta-mee mas-ka?
Where (show me)	見せてください	みせてください	mee-se-te-koo-da-sa-ee
Gone now	もう無いです	もうないです	mo-na-ee-des

Still present	まだ痛みがあります	まだいたみがあります	ma-da-EE-ta-mee-ga-a-ree-mas
Sudden/gradual onset	突然/徐々に	とつぜん/じょじょに	to-tsoo-zen / jo-jo-nee
What bothers you the most?	一番気になっていることは何ですか？	いちばんきになっていることはなんですか	ee-chee-ban kee-nee-nat-te-ee-roo ko-to-wa nan-des-ka
Why did you come today?	今日は何で来たんですか	きょうはなんできたんですか	k-yo-wa-nan-de KEE-tan-des-ka
QUALITY			
If '0' is no pain and 10 is maximum pain, what number do you have now?	痛みの範囲が0−10だとしたらいくつくらいですか。(10が一番痛くて)	いたみのはんいが0−10だとしたらいくつくらいですか	ee-ta-mee-no-han-EE-ga ze-ro ka-ra joo da-to-sheet-a-ra ee-koo-tsoo-koo-ra-EE-de-soo-ka
Burning	燃えるような	もえるような	mo-e-roo-yo-o-na
Constant	不変性な	ふへんせいな	hoo-hen-sey-na
Dull	鈍い	にぶい	nee-boo-ee
Intermittent	痛みに感覚が空きますか？	いたみにかんかくがあきますか	ee-ta-mee-nee-kan-ka-koo-ga-a-kee-mas-ka?
Pressure	圧迫感	あっぱくかん	a-pa-koo-kan
Severe	激しい	はげしい	ha-ge-shee
Sharp/prickly pains	鋭い	するどい	soo-roo-do-ee
Throbbing	動悸	どうき	do-kee
ASSOCIATED SYMPTOMS			
Onset during... (before/after)	この症状はいつからですか	このじょうきょうはいつからですか	ko-no-sho-jo-wa-ee-tsoo-ka-ra-des-ka
Worse (with...)	...で悪化しましたか	...であっかしましたか	...de-at-ka-shee-ma-shee-ta-ka

(cont.)

Better (with...)	...時に楽になりますか	...ときにらくになりますか	...to-kee-nee ra-koo-nee-na-ree-mas-ka
Cough	せき		se-kee
Deep breath	深呼吸	しんこきゅう	sheen-ko-kyoo
Emotional upset	感情的/興奮	かんじょうてき/こうふん	kan-jo-te-kee/ko-hoon
Food	食べ物	たべもの	ta-be-mo-no
Movement	動作	どうさ	do-sa
Nothing	何でも	なんでも	nan-de-mo
Positioning	位置	いち	ee-chee
Rest	休む	やすむ	ya-soo-moo
Walking	歩く	あるく	a-roo-koo

TIME COURSE

For how long?	どれぐらい?		do-re-goo-ra-ee?
Today	今日	きょう	kyo
Yesterday	昨日	きのう	kee-no-oo
How many...	何…	なん	nan...
Months/weeks/days/hours/seconds	ヶ月/週間/日/時間/秒	かげつ/しゅうかん/にち/じかん/びょう	kat-ge-tsoo/shoo-kan/nee-chee/jee-kan/byo
Still present?	まだ痛みは残っていますか?	まだいたみはのこっていますか	ma-da-ee-ta-mee-wa no-kot-te-ee-mas-ka
Gone now?	無くなりましたか?	なくなりましたか	na-koo-na-ree-ma-shee-ta-ka
How long did it last? (See Numbers List)	痛みの期間はどれぐらいでしたか	いたみのきかんはどれぐらいでしたか	ee-ta-mee no kee-kan wa do-re-goo-ra-ee-de-shee-ta-ka
Have you had this before?	前にも似たような事がありましたか	まえにもにたようなことがありましたか	ma-e-nee-mo nee-ta-yo-na-ko-to-ga a-ree-ma-shee-ta-ka

How many times?	何回目ですか？	なんかいめですか？	nan-ka-ee-me-des-ka
When was the last time?	その時はいつでしたか？	そのときはいつでしたか	so-no-to-kee-wa ee-tsoo-de-shee-ta-ka
New	新しい	あたらしい	a-ta-ra-shee
Old	古い	ふるい	hoo-roo-ee
CONTEXT			
Did you...?	あなたは…		a-na-ta-wa...
fall	落ちる	おちる	o-chee-roo?
trip	転ぶ	ころぶ	ko-ro-boo?
faint	気絶する	きぜつする	kee-ze-tsoo-soo-roo?
twist	曲げる/ねんざ	まげる/ねんざ	ma-ge-roo/nen-za?
get hit	打たれる	うたれる	oo-ta-re-roo?
get burned	火傷する	やけどする	ya-ke-do-soo-roo?
get assaulted	殴打される	おうだされる	o-oo-da-sa-re-roo?
get bitten (human/dog/cat/insect)	噛まれる	かまれる	ka-ma-re-roo?
PAST MEDICAL HISTORY			
Take medication?	いつも飲んでいる薬がありますか？	いつものんでいるくすりがありますか	ee-tsoo-mo non-de-ee-roo-koo-soo-ree-ga a-ree-mas-ka?
(aspirin/antibiotics)	アスピリン/抗生物質	あすぴりん/こうせいぶっしつ	a-su-pee-reen / ko-oo-sey-boo-tsoo-shee-tsoo
Do you have (See also Medical Problem List)...	ありますか		a-ree-mas-ka
allergies	アレルギー	あれるぎー	a-re-roo-GEE

(cont.)

medical problems	病歴	びょうれき	byo-re-kee
Do you have problems of the…(see Body Parts List)	…の問題	…のもんだい	…no-MON-da-ee

SURGICAL HISTORY

Have you had surgery?	手術を受けた事はありますか	しゅじゅつをうけたことはありますか	shoo-joo-TSOO wo oo-KE-ta ko-to wa a-ree-mas-ka
Surgery on/"to remove"…(see Body Parts List)	__に手術を受けた事はありますか	__にしゅじゅつをうけたことはありますか	_nee shoo-joo-TSOO wo oo-KE-ta ko-to wa a-ree-mas-ka

SOCIAL HISTORY

Smoke?	タバコは吸いますか？	たばこはすいますか	TA-BA-ko wa soo-ee-mas-ka?
Drink?	お酒を飲みますか？	おさけはのみますか	o-SA-KE wa no mee-mas-ka?
Take drugs?	麻薬は使いますか？	まやくはつかいますか	ma-ya-koo wa TSOO-ka-ee mas-ka?
Recent travel?	最近旅行しましたか？	さいきんりょこうしましたか	SA-ee-keen ryo-KO-oo shee-ma-shee-ta-ka?
Are you sexually active?	最近性行為は行っていますか？	さいきんせいこういはおこなっていますか	SA-ee-keen SEY-ko-ee wa O-KO-nat-te-ee-mas-ka?
Do you use condoms?	コンドームは使いますか？	こんどーむはつかいますか	kon-DO-moo wa TSOO-ka-ee-mas-ka?
Homosexual	ホモセクシャル		ho-MO SE-koo-sha-roo

SYSTEMS REVIEW

Do you have…	__を持っていますか	__をもっていますか	__wo mot-te ee-mas-ka

GENERAL

Fever	熱	ねつ	ne-TSOO

Chills	寒気	さむけ	sa-MOO-ke
Weight loss	体重減少	たいじゅうげんしょう	tay-joo GEN-sho-oo
Fatigue	疲れ	つかれ	TSOO-ka-re
Sick contact	病人との接触	びょうにんとのせっしょく	byo-neen to no se-tsoo-SHO-koo

HEENT

Sore throat	耳鼻科	じびか	jee-bee-ka
Runny nose	鼻水が出ますか	はなみずが出ますか	ha-na-mee-ZOO ga de-mas-ka
Nosebleed	鼻血	はなぢ	ha-NA-jee
Ear pain	中耳炎	ちゅうじえん	CHOO-jee-en
Ear ringing	耳鳴り	みみなり	mee-MEE-na-ree
Decreased hearing	聴力の低下	ちょうりょくのていか	CHO-ryo-koo no tey-ka

EYE

Eye pain	目の痛み	めのいたみ	me no eeTA-mee
Blurry vision	ぼやけ	ぼやけ	BO-ya-ke
Diplopia	複視	ふくし	hoo-KOO-shee
Foreign body sensation	ゴロゴロする		go-ro-go-ro-soo-roo
Contact lenses	コンタクトレンズ		kon-TA-KOO-to ren-zoo

CARDIAC

Chest pain	胸が痛い	むねがいたい	moo-ne-ga ee-ta-ee
Palpitations	心悸亢進	しんきこうしん	sheen-KEE KO-oo-sheen
Orthopnea	起坐呼吸	きざこきゅう	kee-ZA-ko-kyoo
Dyspnea on exertion	無理すると呼吸困難になりますか	むりするときゅうこんなんになりますか	moo-ree SOO-ROO to ko-KYOO-KON-nan nee na-ree-ma-soo-ka

(cont.)

Fainting (syncope)	気を失う	きをうしなう	kee-wo oo-SHEE-na-oo
Leg swelling	足のむくみ	あしのむくみ	a-shee-no MOO-KOO-mee
How many pillows?	枕はいくつ使っていますか？	まくらはいくつつかっていますか	ma-koo-ra wa ee-koo-TSOO TSoo0-kat-te ee-mas-ka?

PULMONARY

Trouble breathing	呼吸困難	こきゅうこんなん	ko-KYOO-kon-nan
SOB	息切れ	いきぎれ	ee-KEE-gee-re
Cough	せき		se-KEE
Sputum	たん		tan
Pain on inspiration	息を吸った時に痛み	いきをすったときにいたみ	ee-KEE wo soot-ta to-KEE nee EE-TA-mee
Hemoptysis	喀血	かっけつ	KA-ke-tsoo

GI

Abdominal pain	腹痛	ふくつう	foo-koo-TSOO
Nausea	吐き気	はきけ	ha-KEE-ke
Vomiting	吐く	はく	ha-KOO
Vomiting blood	血を吐く	ちをはく	chee wo HA-KOO
Coffee ground emesis	コーヒー残渣様の吐物	コーヒーざんさようのとぶつ	ko-hee ZAN-sa-yo-oo no to-boo-tsoo
Anorexia	神経性無食欲症	しんけいせいむしょくしょじょう	sheen-key-sey moo-SHO-koo SHO-oo-jo-oo
Diarrhea	下痢	げり	ge-ree
Difficulty swallowing	物が飲み込みにくい	ものがのみこみにくい	mo-no ga NO-MEE nee-koo-ee
BRBPR	血便	けつべん	KE-TSOO-ben
Melena	黒色便	こくしょくべん	ko-koo-SHO-KOO-ben

Pain after eating	食後の痛み	しょくごのいたみ	SHO-koo-go no ee-ta-mee
Worms	寄生虫	きせいちゅう	kee-SEY-choo
Constipation	痔	じ	jee
GU			
Painful urination	小便の時に痛みを感じる	しょうべんのときにいたみをかんじる	SHO-oo-ben no to-kee-nee EE-TA-mee wo kan-jee-roo
Urgent urination	いきなり小便をしたくなる	いきなりしょうべんをしたくなる	EE-KEE na ree SHO-oo-ben wo shee-ta-koo-na-roo
Frequent urination	頻尿	ひんにょう	HEEN-nyo
Bloody urination	血尿		KE-TSOO-nyo
Discharge: vaginal/penile	ペニス漏出/膣帯下	ペニスろうしゅつ/ちつたいげ	PE-nee-soo ro-oo-SHOO-tsoo/chee-tsoo ta-ee-ge
PSYCH			
Anxiety	緊張		KEEN-cho
Depression	うつ病	うつびょう	oo-TSOO-byo-oo
Suicidal thoughts	自殺を試みた事がある		jee-SA-TSOO wo KO-KO-ro-mee-ta ko-to-ga-a-roo
Homicidal thoughts	他殺を試みた事がある		ta-SA-TSOO wo KO-KO-ro-mee-ta ko-to-ga-a-roo
Medication overdose	過剰摂取	かじょうせっしゅ	ka-jo-oo se-SHOO
Hear voices	声が聞こえる	こえがきこえる	ko-e ga KEE-KO-e-roo
NEURO			
Headache	頭痛	ずつう	zoo-TSO-OO

(cont.)

Japanese—日本語

Worst headache of life	人生で一番辛い頭痛	じんせいでいちばんつらいずつう	jeen-sey-de EE-chee-BAN tsoo-ra-ee zoo-TSO-OO
Weakness	弱く	よわく	yo-WA-koo
Dizzy	目まい	めまい	me-ma-ee
What is your name?	貴方のお名前は何ですか？	あなたのおなまえはなんですか？	a-na-ta-no O-na-ma-e wa nan-des-ka?
Where are we?	今何処に居ますか？	いまどこにいますか？	ee-ma-do-KO-nee ee-mas-ka?
What is the year/month/date?	今日は何月何日ですか	きょうはなんがつなんにちですか	kyo-wa nan-GA-tsoo nan-nee-chee des-ka?
Bowel dysfunction	腸管機能不全	ちょうかんきのうふぜん	CHO-oo-kan kee-no-oo hoo-zen
Bladder dysfunction	神経因性膀胱	しんけいいんせいぼうこう	sheen-key EEN-sey bo-oo-ko-oo
Photophobia	まぶしがり		ma-BOO-shee-ga-ree
Tingling/numbness	しびれる		shee-bee-re-roo
Decreased strength in... (See Body Parts List)	__が弱く感じる	__がよわくかんじる	_ga yo-wa koo kan-jee-roo
Seizure	発作	ほっさ	HOH-sa
Difficulty walking	歩行困難	ほこうこんなん	ho-KO-oo kon-nan
Difficulty speaking	言葉が不明瞭	ことばがふめいりょう	ko-to-BA-ga HOO-mey-ryo
Spinning (vertigo)	くらくらする		koo-ra-koo-ra-soo-roo
Confusion	混乱	こんらん	kon-ran
MISC			
Lump	しこり		shee-ko-ree

Itching	かゆい		ka-yoo-ee
Bruising	あざ		aza
Rash	皮疹	ひしん	hee-sheen
Swelling	はれ物	はれもの	ha-re-mo-no
Jaundice (yellow skin)	黄疸	おうだん	O-oo-dan

GYNECOLOGIC

Vaginal bleeding	膣から出血	ちつからしゅっけつ	CHEE-tsoo ka-ra shoo-ke-tsoo
Heavy	多量	たりょう	ta-ryo
Irregular	不定期	ふていき	HOO-tey-kee
Absent	不在	ふざい	HOO-za-ee
Vaginal discharge	膣帯下	ちつたいか	CHEE-TSOO ta-ee-ka
Pelvic pain	腰痛	ようつう	YO-oo-tsoo
Rape	レイプ		REY-poo
Pain with intercourse	性行為の時に痛み		sey-KO-oo-ee no TO-KEE nee ee-ta-mee
Contraceptive	避妊薬	ひにんやく	HEE-neen-ya-koo

OBSTETRIC

Are you pregnant?	妊娠していますか	にんしんしていますか	NEEN-sheen shee-te ee-mas-ka?
LMP how many days ago?	最後の生理はいつですか	さいごのせいりはいつですか	SA-ee-go no SEY-ree wa ee-tsoo-des-ka?
Times pregnant?	妊娠の回数は何ですか？	にんしんのかいすうはなんですか	NEEN-sheen no ka-ee-soo wa nan-des-ka?
Times delivered?	出産の回数は何ですか？	しゅっさんのかいすうはなんですか	SHOO-san no ka-EE-soo wa nan-des-ka?
Miscarriage	流産	りゅうざん	ryoo-zan

(cont.)

Abortion	流産	りゅうざん	ryoo-zan
Fluid leakage	破水	はすい	HA-soo-ee
Contraction	筋肉が収れん	きんにくがしゅうれん	keen-NEE-koo ga shoo-ren
Fetal movement	胎児が動く	たいじがうごく	ta-EE-jee ga oo-go-koo

TRAUMA

How many hours ago did you eat last?	食事は何時間前に取りましたか	しょくじはなんじかんまえにとりましたか	sho-KOO-jee wa nan-JEE-kan ma-e-nee-TO-ree ma-shee-ta-ka?
Lost consciousness?	気絶しましたか？	きぜつしましたか	kee-ze-TSOO shee-ma-shee-ta-ka?
Tetanus within 5 years?	5年以内に破傷風はありましたか	5ねんいないにはしょうふうはありましたか	go-nen ee-na-ee-nee HA-SHO-hoo wa a-ree-ma-shee-ta-ka?

PEDIATRIC

How old?	何歳ですか	なんさいですか	nan-sa-EE des-ka?
Vaccines up to date?	ワクチンを全部摂取しましたか	わくちんをぜんぶせっしゅしましたか	wa-koo-CHEEN wo zen-boo SEH-shoo shee-ma-shee-ta-ka?
Urinating normally	普通に尿が出ますか	ふつうににょうがでますか	hoo-TSOO nee nyo ga de-mas-ka
Taking liquids	水分摂取していますか	すいぶんせっしゅしていますか	soo-EE-boon SEH-shoo shee-te-ee-mas-ka
Increased crying	泣く回数が増えていますか？	なくかいすうがふえていますか	nak-oo ka-ee-soo ga HOO-e-te ee-mas-ka
Ingestion	食物摂取	しょくもつせっしゅ	SHO-koo-mo-tsoo SEH-shoo
Foreign body	異物	いぶつ	ee-boo-tsoo
Premature	早産	そうざん	so-oo-zan

Birth complications	出産困難	しゅっさんこんなん	SHOO-san kon-nan
PHYSICAL EXAM/INSTRUCTION			
Sit down (please)	座って下さい	すわってください	soo-WAT-te koo-da-sa-ee
Lie down	仰向けになって下さい	あおむけになってください	a-o-MOO-KE-nee nat-te koo-da-sa-ee
Come here	こちらに来て下さい	こちらにきてください	ko-CHEE-ra nee kee-te koo-da-sa-ee
Relax	リラックスして下さい	りらっくすしてください	ree-rah-KOO-soo shee-te-koo-da-sa-ee
Don't move	動かないで下さい	うごかないでください	oo-go-KA-na-ee de koo-da-sa-ee
Open your mouth	口を開けて下さい	くちをあけてください	koo-CHEE wo a-ke-te koo-da-sa-ee
Say "ahh"	「アー」と言って下さい	「あー」といってください	aaa to ee-te koo-da-sa-ee
Swallow	飲み込んで下さい	のみこんでください	no-mee-KON-de koo-da-sa-ee
Breath deeply	深呼吸をして下さい	しんこきゅうをしてください	sheen-ko-KYOO wo shee-te-koo-da-sa-ee
Hold your breath	息を止めて下さい	いきをとめてください	ee-kee wo to-me-te koo-da-sa-ee
Cough	せき		se-kee
Push	押して下さい	おしてください	O-SHEE-te koo-da-sa-ee
Pull	引っ張って下さい	ひっぱってください	hee-pat-te koo-da-sa-ee
Follow my finger	指を追って下さい	ゆびをおってください	yoo-bee wo ot-te koo-da-sa-ee
Close your eyes	目を閉じて下さい	めをとじてください	me wo to-jee-te koo-da-sa-ee
Smile	緊張しないでください	きんちょうしないでください	KEEN-cho-oo shee-na-ee-de koo-da-sa-ee

(cont.)

134 Japanese—日本語

Can you feel this?	これを感じますか？	これをかんじますか	ko-re wo KAN-jee mas-ka
Copy this (movement)	私の動きの通りにしてみてください	わたしのうごきのとおりにしてみてください	wa-ta-shee no oo-go-kee no to-oo-ree nee shee te-mee-te-koo-da-sa-ee
I am going to put a finger in your rectum	腸の触診をします	ちょうのちょくしん	choo-oo no CHO-koo-sheen
I am going to examine your vagina	膣を触診します	ちつをちょくしん	chee-tsoo wo cho-koo-sheen

REASSESSMENT

Do you feel better?	良くなりましたか？	よくなりましたか	yo-koo-na-ree ma-shee-ta-ka?
Do you feel worse?	悪化しましたか？	あっかしましたか	AH-ka shee-ma-shee-ta-ka?

PATIENT WORDS

I hurt	痛いです	いたいです	ee-ta-ee de-soo
Help!	助けて！	たすけて！	ta-SOO-ke-te!
Bathroom	トイレ		to-ee-re
Food	食べ物	たべもの	ta-be-mo-no
Water	水	みず	mee-zoo

PROCEDURES & CONSENT

You need...	__が必要です	__がひつようです	_ga-hee-tsoo-yo-oo-des
Injection	注入	ちゅうにゅう	CHOO-nyoo
Stiches	縫う	ぬう	noo-oo
Cast	ギブス		GEE-boo-soo
Crutches	松葉杖	まつばうづえ	ma-tsoo-ba-zoo-e
Perform surgery on the... (See Body Parts List)	__に手術	__にしゅじゅつ	_nee-shoo-joo-tsoo

The risks are...	リスクは		ree-soo-koo-wa
Bleeding	出血	しゅっけつ	SHOOT-ke-tsoo
Infection	感染	かんせん	kan-sen
Scar	傷跡	きずあと	kee-zoo-A-TO
Repeat procedure	もう一回やります	もういっかいやります	mo-oo-EE-KA-EE ya-ree-ma-soo
Iodine	ヨウ素	ようそ	yo-oo-so
Damage to your...(See Body Parts List)	__に損害	__にそんがい	_nee-son-ga-ee
Sign here	サインして下さい	サインしてください	sa-een-shee-te-koo-da-sa-ee
TESTS			
X-ray	エックス線	エックスせん	et-KOO-SOO-sen
C.A.T. Scan	CTスキャン		shee-tee-soo-kyan
Ultrasound	超音波診断	ちょうおんぱしんだん	cho-oo-on-pa sheen-dan
Catheterization/ bladder catheter	カテーテル/導尿管	どうにょうかん	ka-te-te-roo/do-oo-nyo-kan
Colonoscopy (from below)/ Endoscopy (from above)	大腸内視鏡	だいちょうないしきょう	da-ee-cho-oo na-ee-shee-kyo
Endoscopy	内視鏡	ないしきょう	na-ee-shee-KYO
END OF LIFE			
Do you want us to...	__を私達にして欲しいですか	__をわたしたちにしてほしいですか	_wo wa-ta-shee ta-chee-nee shee-te-ho-shee des-ka
Perform CPR	心肺機能蘇生を行って下さい	しんぱいきのうそせい	sheen-pa-ee kee-no-oo so-sey

(cont.)

Defibrillate	除細動	じょさいどう	JO-sa-ee-do-oo
Intubate	喉に管を差込む	のどにかんをさしこむ	no-do-nee kan wo sa-shee-ko-moo
He/she is dead	お亡くなりになりました	おなくなりになりました	O-NA-koo-na-ree nee-na-ree-ma-shee-ta
We did all we could	出来る限りの事をしました	できるかぎりのことをしました	de-kee-roo ka-gee-ree no ko-to wo shee-ma shee-ta

DISCHARGE

You have...(See Medical Prob List)	貴方は__を抱えています	あなたは__をかかえています	a-na-ta wa _ wo KA-KA-e-te ee-mas
He/she is going to stay in the hospital	彼/彼女を入院させます	彼/彼女を入院させます	ka-re / ka-no-jo wo nyoo-een-sa-se-mas
Take "X" pills "Y" times a day for "Z" days	"Z"日間の間に"X"条薬を一日に"Y"回 飲んでください	"Z"にちかんのあいだに"X"じょくすりをいちにちに"Y"かい のんでください	"Z" nichi -kan no a-ee-da-nee "X" jo-koo-soo-ree wo ee-chee-nee-chee-nee "Y" kai non-de-koo-da-sa-ee
Pills	ピル		pee-roo
Antibiotics	抗生物質	こうせいぶっしつ	ko-oo-sey boo-SHEE-tsoo
Before/after meals	食前/食後	しょくぜん/しょくご	SHO-KOO-zen / SHO-KOO-go
Return to the ER if...	何かあったらERに戻って来て下さい	なにかあったらERにもどってきてください	na-nee-KA AT-ta-ra ER nee-MO-DOT-TE KEE-TE koo-da-sa-ee
Follow up at "X" on "Y"	"X"で"Y"の事に関して尋ねてください	"X"で"Y"のことにかんしてたずねてください	"X" de "Y" no-koto-nee kan-shee-te TA-ZOO-NE-Te-koo-da-sa-ee
You're welcome	どいたしまして		do-EE-TA-shee ma-shee-te
Goodbye	さようなら		sa-yo-oo-na-ra

MEDICAL PROBS			
AIDS/HIV	エイズ/HIV		e-ee-zoo/e-ee-chee a-ee vee
Anemia	貧血症	ひんけつしょう	heen-KE-TSOO-sho-oo
Arrhythmia	不整脈	ふせいみゃく	hoo-sey-MYA-koo
Arthritis	関節炎	かんせつえん	kan-SE-TSOO-en
Asthma	ぜんそく		zen-so-koo
Bronchitis	気管支炎	きかんしえん	kee-KAN-shee-en
Cancer	癌	がん	gan
Cirrhosis	肝硬変	かんこうへん	kan-KO-oo-hen
Cholesterol	コレステロール		ko-re-soo-te-ro-roo
Cold	風邪	かぜ	ka-ze
Constipation	便秘	べんぴ	ben-PEE
Cyst	嚢腫	のうしゅ	no-oo-shoo
Diabetes	糖尿病	とうにょうびょう	to-oo-NYO-oo- byo
Dialysis	透析	とうせき	to-oo-se-KEE
Diverticulitis	憩室炎	けいしつえん	key-shee-TSOO-en
Emphysema	気腫	きほう	KEE-ho-oo
Fibroids	子宮筋腫	しきゅうきんしゅ	shee-kyoo keen-shoo
Fracture	骨折	こっせつ	KOH-se-tsoo
Flu	インフルエンザ		een-hoo-roo en-za
Gallstones	胆石	たんせき	tan-se-kee
Gastritis/GERD	胃炎/胃食道逆流症	いえん	EE-en
Hepatitis	肝炎	かんえん	kan-en
Heart attack	心臓発作	しんぞうほっさ	SHEEN-zo-oo HOT-sa

(cont.)

Heart disease	心臓病	しんぞうびょう	SHEEN-zo-oo-byo
Heart failure	心不全	ふしんぜん	hoo-SHEEN-zen
Hypertension	高血圧	こうけつあつ	ko-oo-KE-TSOO-a-tsoo
Indigestion	消化不良	しょうかふりょう	sho-oo-KA hoo-ryo
Kidney stone	尿路結石	にょうろけっせき	NYO-oo-ro keh-se-kee
Lupus	全身性エリテマトーデス	ぜんしんせいえりてまとーです	ZEN-sheen-sey e-ree-te-ma to-des
Migraine	偏頭痛	へんとうつう	hen-to-tsoo
Murmur	雑音	ざつおん	ZA-TSOO-on
Pacemaker	ペースメーカー		pey-soo-mey-kaa
Pneumonia	肺炎	はいえん	hay-en
Seizures	発作	ほっさ	HOH-sa
STD	性病気	せいびょうき	sey-byo-oo-kee
Stroke	発作	はっさ	HAH-sa
Ulcer	潰瘍	かいよう	ka-ee-yo-oo
Ulcerative colitis	潰瘍性大腸炎	かいようせいだいちょうえん	ka-ee-yo-oo sey-da-ee-cho-en
UTI	尿路感染症	にょうろかんせんしょう	nyo-oo-ro kan-sen sho
BODY PARTS			
Abdomen	お腹	おなか	O-NA-ka
Ankle	足首	あしくび	a-shee-koo-bee
Appendix	盲腸	もうちょう	mo-oo-cho-oo
Arm	腕	うで	oo-de
Artery	血管	けっかん	KET-kan
Back	背中	せなか	SE-na-ka

Japanese—日本語

Bladder	膀胱	ぼうこう	bo-oo-ko-oo
Blood	血	ち	chee
Bone	骨	ほね	ho-ne
Brain	脳	のう	no-oo
Breast	乳	ちち	chee-chee
Calf	ふくらはぎ		hoo-koo-ra-ha-gee
Chest	胸	むね	moo-ne
Chin	あご		a-go
Ear	耳	みみ	mee-mee
Elbow	肱	ひじ	hee-jee
Eye	目	め	me
Face	顔	かお	ka-o
Finger	指	ゆび	yoo-bee
Foot	足	あしくび	a-shee-koo-bee
Hand	手	て	te
Head	頭	あたま	a-TA-ma
Heart	心臓	しんぞう	sheen-zo-oo
Gallbladder	胆嚢	のう	no-oo
Jaw	あご		a-go
Joint	間接	かんせつ	kan-se-tsoo
Kidney	腎臓	じんぞう	jeen-zo-oo
Knee	膝	ひざ	hee-za
Leg	脚	あし	a-shee
Liver	肝臓	かんぞう	kan-zo-oo
Mouth	口	くち	koo-chee
Muscle	筋肉	きんにく	keen-nee-koo

(cont.)

Neck	首	くび	koo-bee
Nerve	神経	しんけい	sheen-KEY
Nose	鼻	はな	ha-na
Ovary	卵巣	らんそう	ran-so-oo
Pancreas	膵臓	ひぞう	hee-zo-oo
Penis	ペニス	ぺにす	PE-nee-soo
Prostate	前立腺	ぜんりつせん	ZEN-ree-tsoo-sen
Rectum	直腸	ちょくちょう	cho-KOO-cho
Rib	肋骨	ろっこつ	rot-KO-TSOO
Shoulder	肩	かた	ka-ta
Skin	皮膚	ひふ	hee-hoo
Spleen	脾臓	ひぞう	hee-zo-oo
Spine	背骨	せぼね	SE-BO-ne
Stomach	お腹	おなか	O-NA-ka
Teeth	歯	は	ha
Testicle	精巣	せいそう	sey-so-oo
Throat	喉	のど	no-do
Thyroid	甲状腺	こうじょうせん	ko-oo-jo sen
Toe	手足	てあし	te-a-shee
Tonsils	扁桃腺	へんとうせん	hen-to-sen
Tongue	舌	した	shee-ta
Uterus	子宮	しかん	shee-kan
Vagina	膣	ちつ	chee-tsoo
Vein	静脈	じょうみゃく	jo-mya-koo
Wrist	手首	てくび	te-koo-bee
NUMBERS			
How many (times)?	何回？	なんかい？	nan-ka-ee?

Japanese—日本語

0	ゼロ	ぜろ	ze-ro
1	一	いち	ee-chee
2	二	に	nee
3	三	さん	san
4	四	よん	yon
5	五	ご	go
6	六	ろく	ro-koo
7	七	しち	shee-chee
8	八	はち	ha-chee
9	九	きゅう	kyoo
10	十	じゅう	joo
11	十一	じゅういち	joo-ee-chee
20	二十	にじゅう	nee-joo
30	三十	さんじゅう	san-joo
40	四十	よんじゅう	yon-joo
50	五十	ごじゅう	go-joo
60	六十	ろくじゅう	ro-koo-joo
70	七十	ななじゅう	na-na-joo
80	八十	はちじゅう	ha-chee-joo
90	九十	きゅうじゅう	kyoo-joo
100	百	ひゃく	hee-ya-koo

Korean—한국어

WORD/PHRASE	TRANSLATION	ENGLISH PRONUNCIATION
Korean	언어	han-goo-gu
INTRODUCTION & REGISTRATION		
Hello	안녕하세요	an-NYUNG ha-se-yo
I am a doctor / nurse *(add your name)*	저는 _____의사 _____간호사 입니다	dok-tor ___/gan-ho-sa ___ ip-nee-da
What is your name?	이름이 뭐예요?	ee-rum?
Who is your doctor?	담당의사는 누구세요?	joo-chee-ee ga noo-goo-se-yo?
How old are you?	몇살이세요?	MYUT-sal ee-se-yo?
Birthdate?	생일?	seng-eel?
Telephone number?	전화번호?	jun-hwa-bun-ho?
Address?	주소?	joo-so?
Social security number?	소셜넘버?	so-syal bun-ho?
Insurance?	보험?	bo-hum?
BASICS		
Do you understand?	이해 합니까?	ee-he ha-se-yo?
Yes	네	ne
No	아니오	a-nee-o
Please	부탁합니다	boo-TAK he-yo
Thank you	감사합니다	GAM-sa hap-nee-da
Sorry	죄송합니다 / 미안합니다	mee-an hap-nee-da
I don't understand	이해 못 합니다.	ee-he MOT hap-nee-da
Repeat	다시 한번	DA-shee

(cont.)

Speak slowly	천천히 말씀하세요	chun-chun-hee mal-ha-se-yo
Answer "yes" or "no"	네' 아니면 '아니오' 라고 대답하세요	"ne" a-ni-myun "a-nee-o" de-DAP ha-se-yo
Here	여기	YU-gee
This	이거	ee-gu
It's alright (consoling)	괜찮습니다	gwen chan-a-yo
I'll be right back	다시 오겠습니다	da-shee o-GET sup-nee-da

GENERAL

What's wrong?	무슨 일이 십니까?	moo-soon- eel ee-se-yo?
Pain	고통 / 아픔	go-tong / a-poom
Do you have pain?	아프시나요? 고통을 느끼시나요?	a-poo-se-yo?
Does the pain radiate?	고통이 퍼지는 느낌인가요?	a-poon-gut ee pu-jee-na-yo?
Where (show me)	어디인지 가르켜 주세요	u-dee in-jee bo-yo joo-se-yo
Gone now	이제 없어졌나요? / 이제 없어졌어요.	ee-je UP-na-yo?
Still present	아직 있나요?	a-jik it-na-yo?
Sudden/gradual onset	갑자기 / 조금씩 시작	GAP-ja-gee/chun-chun-hee shee-jak
What bothers you the most?	무엇이 가장 힘든가요?	je-eel him-dun-gut
Why did you come today?	오늘 오신 이유는?	o-nul W-HE o-shut-na-yo?

QUALITY		
If '0' is no pain and 10 is maximum pain, what number do you have now?	만약 '0'이 아프지 않다 '10'이 가장 아픈것이라면 현재 넘버가 뭔가요?	man-yak e "gong(0)" ee an-a-poom/ "ship(10)" ee ga-jang a-poom ee-myon jee-gum moo-sun number in-ga-yo?
Burning	끓는 느낌 / 타는 느낌	TA-nun nu-kim
Constant	지속적	ge-SOK
Dull	무디다	moo-dee-da
Intermittent	때때로	ga-KUM
Pressure	압력	ap-ryuk
Severe	심하다	shim-ha-da
Sharp/prickly pains	날카롭다 / 따끔하다	nal-ka-rop-da/ ta-kum ha-da
Throbbing	두근두근하다	doo-goon doo-goon ha-da
ASSOCIATED SYMPTOMS		
Onset during… (before/after)	증상이 온 시기는? 전에, 후에, 사이에?	JUN-e/ HOO-e shee-jak…
Worse (with…)	더 나빠졌다 (함께…)	na-pa jee-da…
Better (with…)	더 좋아졌다 (함께…)	jo-a jee-da…
Cough	기침	gee-CHIM
Deep breath	심호흡	shim-ho-hup
Emotional upset	정신적 충격	jung-shin choong-gyuk
Food	음식	um-shik
Movement	움직임 / 운동 / 이동	oon-dong/ oom-jee-gim

(cont.)

Nothing	아무것도 없다 / 아무것도 아니다	UP-da/ a-nee-da
Positioning	위치하다	wee-chee ha-da
Rest	쉬다	shee-da
Walking	걷다	gut-da
TIME COURSE		
For how long?	얼마나 오래?	UR-ma-na o-re?
Today	오늘	o-nul
Yesterday	어제	U-je
How many...	얼마나...?	UR-ma-na/ MYUT- ge...?
Months/weeks/days/hours/seconds	달 / 주 / 일 / 시간 / 초	dal/joo/eel/shee-gan/cho
Still present?	아직도 있나요?	a-jik-do it-na-yo?
Gone now?	지금은 없어졌나요?	jee-kum up-su-yo?
How long did it last? (See Numbers List)	얼마나 있었나요?	UR-ma-na o-re IT-SUT-na-yo?
Have you had this before?	이 증상이 전에도 있었나요?	jun-e-do IT-SUT-na-yo?
How many times?	얼마나?	MYUT-bun?
When was the last time?	이 증상이 최근에 있었던 때는 언제였나요?	ma-ji-mak UN-je IT-SUT-na-yo?
New	새로운	se-ro-oon
Old	옛날	o-re/yet-nal
CONTEXT		
Did you...?	다음과 같은 일이 있으셨나요?	(see full phrase below)
fall	넘어지다	num-u JYUT-na-yo?
trip	걸려 넘어지다	gur-ryo num-u-JYUT-na-yo?

faint	기절하다 / 졸도하다	gee-jul ha-shut-na-yo?
twist	꼬이다, 비틀리다	bee-tu-lee-shut-na-yo?
get hit	맞다 / 다치다	ma-JYUT-na-yo?
get burned	화상을 입다	hwa-sang ee-bun-na-yo?
get assaulted	폭행당하다	po-KENG dang-het-na-yo?
get bitten (human/dog/cat/insect)	물리다	mool- lee shut-na-yo?
PAST MEDICAL HISTORY		
Take medication?	약을 드시나요?	YAK du-shee-na-yo?
(aspirin/antibiotics)	(아스피린 / 항생제)	as-pi-rin / hang-seng-je
Do you have (See also Medical Problem List)…	다음과 같은 증상이 있나요?	it-na-yo?
allergies	알레르기	al-le-ru-gi
medical problems	과거의 병역은?	byung-yuk IT-na-yo?
Do you have problems of the… (see Body Parts List)	…신체부위 문제	…shin-che moon-je
SURGICAL HISTORY		
Have you had surgery?	수술 하신 적이 있나요?	soo-sool ha-shin-juk it-na-yo?
Surgery on/"to remove"…(see Body Parts List)	…에 수술을	soo-sool boo-wee / soo-sool han-got…
SOCIAL HISTORY		
Smoke?	흡연을 하시나요?	dam-ba-e ha-se-yo?
Drink?	술을 드시나요?	sool ha-se-yo?

(cont.)

Take drugs?	마약을 복용하시나요?	ma-yak ha-se-yo?
Recent travel?	최근에 여행을 하셨나요?	yu-heng ha-SHUT-na-yo?
Are you sexually active?	성 관계는 가지시나요?	sex ha-se-yo?
Do you use condoms?	콘돔을 사용하시나요?	condom sa-yong ha-se-yo?
Homosexual	동성애	dong-sung-a-e

SYSTEMS REVIEW

Do you have...	이런 증상이 있나요...?	IT-na-yo...?

GENERAL

Fever	열	yul
Chills	오한	o-han
Weight loss	체중 감소	che-joong gam-so
Fatigue	피로	pee-ro
Sick contact	주위에 아픈 분	joo-wee e a-poon-boon

HEENT

Sore throat	인후염 / 목이 아프다	mok a-poo-da
Runny nose	콧물이 흐른다	KOT-mool
Nosebleed	코피가 난다	ko-pee
Ear pain	귀가 아프다	gwee a-poo-da
Ear ringing	귀에서 윙윙 소리가 난다	gwee e so-ree nan-da
Decreased hearing	청각감소	CHUNG-gak gam-so

EYE

Eye pain	눈이 아프다	noon a-poo-da
Blurry vision	흐릿하게 보인다	jal an-bo-in-da

Diplopia	물체가 두개로 보인다	doo-ge-ro bo-in-da
Foreign body sensation	이물질 느낌	e-mool-jil nu-kim
Contact lenses	콘택트 렌즈	con-tac-t len-z
CARDIAC		
Chest pain	가슴이 아프다	ga-sum a-poo-da
Palpitations	가슴이 두근거린다	ga-sum doo-koon gu-rin-da
Orthopnea	호흡곤란	ho-hup go-lan
Dyspnea on exertion	숨을 내쉴때 곤란하다	oon-dong hal-te ho-hup go-lan
Fainting (syncope)	기절	gee-jul
Leg swelling	다리가 붓는다	da-ree boo-oom
How many pillows?	베개를 몇개?	byo-ge MYUT-ge sa-yong ha-se-yo?
PULMONARY		
Trouble breathing	호흡곤란	ho-hup go-lan
SOB	숨차다	soom cha-da
Cough	기침	gee-chim
Sputum	가래	ga-re
Pain on inspiration	숨을 들이킬때 곤란하다	soom shil-te him-dul-da
Hemoptysis	기도 또는 폐에서 혈액을 토한다	pee to-han-da
GI		
Abdominal pain	복부에 고통이 있다	be a-poom
Nausea	메스껍다	me-soo ku-oom
Vomiting	구토	goo-to

(cont.)

Vomiting blood	피를 토하다	pee to-ha-da
Coffee ground emesis	커피색 토하다	ko-fee SEK to-ha-da
Anorexia	식욕부진	shee-GYOK-boo-jin
Diarrhea	설사	SUL-sa
Difficulty swallowing	음식을 삼키기 어렵다	um-shik sam-kee-gee him-dul-da
BRBPR	항문에 피가 보인다	hang-moon-e pee-ga bo-in-da
Melena	하혈	ha-hyol
Pain after eating	음식을 먹고난 후 아프다	muk-go-nan-hoo a-poo-da
Worms	회충	h-we-choong
Constipation	변비	byon-bee
GU		
Painful urination	소변 볼때 아프다	so-byun a-poo-da
Urgent urination	소변이 갑자기 마렵다	so-byun gap-ja-gee ma-ryup-da
Frequent urination	소변을 자주 본다	so-byun ja-joo bon-da
Bloody urination	소변에 피가 있다	so-byun-e pee-it-da
Discharge: vaginal/penile	질/피너스 분비물	jeel/pe-nis boon-bee-mool
PSYCH		
Anxiety	불안하다	boo-lan ha-da
Depression	우울증	oo-wool-jung
Suicidal thoughts	자살충동	ja-sal ha-go-sip-da
Homicidal thoughts	살인충동	sa-rin ha-go-sip-da
Medication overdose	약 과잉복용	YAK gua-ing bo-gyong
Hear voices	목소리가 들린다	MOK-so-ree dul-lin-da

NEURO		
Headache	두통	doo-tong
Worst headache of life	겪어본 중 세상에서 가장 아픈 두통	je-eel a-poon doo-tong
Weakness	허약함	hu-YAK
Dizzy	어지러움증	u-jee-ru-oom
What is your name?	이름이 뭡니까?	ee-rum?
Where are we?	우리가 어디에 있지요?	yu-gee u-dee-jee-yo?
What is the year/month/date?	오늘이 몇년도 몇월 몇일 이지요?	o-nul MYUT-nyon MYUT-cheel?
Bowel dysfunction	내장 기능장애	ne-jang jang-e
Bladder dysfunction	방광 기능장애	so-byon jang-e
Photophobia	빛 공포증	bit gong-po-jung
Tingling/numbness	욱신거리다 / 무감각	moo-gam-gak
Decreased strength in...(See Body Parts List)	체력감소	YAK-he-jee-da
Seizure	간질	gan-jeel
Difficulty walking	걷는게 힘든다	gu-rum him-dul-da
Difficulty speaking	말할때 힘든다	mal hal-te him-dul-da
Spinning (vertigo)	현기증	u-jee-ru-oom/ hyon-gee-jung
Confusion	정신착란	jung-shin chak-lan
MISC		
Lump	덩어리 / 혹	dung-u-ree/ hok
Itching	가렵다	ga-ryo-oom
Bruising	멍들다	mung

(cont.)

Rash	발진 / 뽀루지	bal-jin
Swelling	붓다	boo-um
Jaundice (yellow skin)	황달	hwang-dal
GYNECOLOGIC		
Vaginal bleeding	질 출혈	jeel chool-hyul
Heavy	양이 많다	yang ee man-ta
Irregular	불규칙하다	bool gyu-chik
Absent	거르다	up-da
Vaginal discharge	질 분비물	jeel boon-bee-mool
Pelvic pain	골반에 고통이 있다	gol-ban a-poom
Rape	강간 당하다	gang-gan
Pain with intercourse	섹스 할 때 아픔	sex hal-te a-poom
Contraceptive	피임	pee-im
OBSTETRIC		
Are you pregnant?	임신중 입니까?	im-shin-joong ee-se-yo?
LMP how many days ago?	마지막 생리	ma-jee-mak seng-lee?
Times pregnant?	임신 횟수	im-shin MYUT-bun het-su-yo?
Times delivered?	출산 횟수	chool-san MYUT-bun het-su-yo?
Miscarriage	유산	yoo-san
Abortion	임신중절	im-shin joong-jul
Fluid leakage	양수 누출	yang-soo noo-chool
Contraction	수축	soo-chook
Fetal movement	태아의 움직임	te-a oom-jee-gim

Korean—한국어

TRAUMA		
How many hours ago did you eat last?	몇시간전에 식사를 하셨나요?	ma-jee-mak shik-sa un-je ha-shut-na-yo?
Lost consciousness?	정신을 잃으셨나요?	jung-shin ee-ru-shut-na-yo?
Tetanus within 5 years?	마지막 파상풍 주사	ma-jee-mak p a-sang-poong joo-sa?
PEDIATRIC		
How old?	몇살이에요?	a-e-gee myut-sal?
Vaccines up to date?	예방접종은 다 맞혔나요 ?	ye-bang-jup-jong?
Urinating normally	소변은 정상적으로 보나요?	so-byun jung-sang in-ga-yo?
Taking liquids	액체류를 섭취하고 있나요?	ma-shil-soo it-na-yo?
Increased crying	더 많이 우나요?	du ma-nee u-na-yo?
Ingestion	섭취	sup-ch-wee
Foreign body	이물질	ee-mool-jil
Premature	미숙아	mee-soo-ga
Birth complications	출산의 어려움	chool-san u-ryu-oom
PHYSICAL EXAM/INSTRUCTION		
Sit down (please)	앉으세요	an-z-se-yo
Lie down	누우세요	noo-oo-se-yo
Come here	이쪽으로 오세요	ee-ree o-se-yo
Relax	편하게 계세요	pyun-ha-ge ge-se-yo
Don't move	움직이지 마세요	oom-jee-gee-jee ma-se-yo
Open your mouth	입을 벌리세요	ip bul-ee-se-yo
Say "ahh"	아' 하세요	"a" ha-se-yo

(cont.)

Swallow	삼키세요	sam-kee-se-yo
Breath deeply	호흡을 깊게 들이세요	soom gip-ge shwee-se-yo
Hold your breath	숨을 잡고 계세요	soom cham-u-se-yo
Cough	기침을 하세요	gee-chim ha-se-yo
Push	미세요	mee-se-yo
Pull	당기세요	dang-gee-se-yo
Follow my finger	제 손가락을 따라 오세요	je son-ka-rak bo-se-yo
Close your eyes	눈을 감으세요	noon gam-u-se-yo
Smile	웃어보세요	woo-su bo-se-yo
Can you feel this?	이걸 느끼세요?	noo-kee-se-yo?
Copy this (movement)	따라하세요	T-HA-ra ha-se-yo
I am going to put a finger in your rectum	항문검사 합니다	hang-moon gum-sa hap-nee-da
I am going to examine your vagina	질검사 합니다	jeel gum-sa hap-nee-da

REASSESSMENT

Do you feel better?	더 좋아 졌나요?	jo-a JYUT-na-yo?
Do you feel worse?	더 나빠 졌나요?	na-pa JYUT-na-yo?

PATIENT WORDS

I hurt	아파요	a-pa-yo
Help!	도와주세요	do-wa joo-se-yo
Bathroom	화장실	hwa-jang-shil
Food	음식	um-shik/ bap
Water	물	mool

PROCEDURES & CONSENT		
You need...	_____ 필요합니다	___ pee-ryo hap-nee-da
Injection	주사	joo-sa
Stiches	꿰메야 합니다	ko-me-ya hap-nee-da
Cast	캐스팅	kes-ting
Crutches	목발	mok-bal
Perform surgery on the... (See Body Parts List)	다음 _____ 에 수술을 합니다	___ soo-sool hap-nee-da
The risks are...	다음과 같은 위험이 있습니다	ee-run wee-hum it-sup-nee-da
Bleeding	출혈	chool-hyul
Infection	감염	gam yom
Scar	흉터	hyoong-tu
Repeat procedure	_____ 반복	da-shee
Iodine	요오디	yo-o-d
Damage to your... (See Body Parts List)	손상 (신체부위)	son-sang (shin-che boo-wee)
Sign here	여기에 서명을 하세요	sign (su-myong) ha-se-yo
TESTS		
X-ray	엑스-레이	x-rey
C.A.T. Scan	커퓨터 X선 체축 단층 촬영사진 (CT 스켄)	see-tee ch-wal-yong
Ultrasound	초음파	cho-oom-pa
Catheterization/ bladder catheter	도뇨관 (카터터) 설치 (삽입)	ka-te-tu sap-ip

(cont.)

Colonoscopy (from below)/Endoscopy (from above)	결장경 검사	gyol-jang-gyong gum-sa
Endoscopy	내시경 검사	ne-shee-gyung gum-sa

END OF LIFE

Do you want us to...	저희가 _____하길 원하십니까?	_____ha-gil won-ha-se-yo?
Perform CPR	심폐기능소생법을 합니다	shim-pe so-seng hap-nee-da
Defibrillate	세동을 멈추다	se-dong mum-choo-da/ de-fib-ril-leyt
Intubate	삽관 치료	sap-gwan chee-ryo
He/she is dead	운명하셨습니다 / 죽었습니다	dol-a ga-shut-sup-nee-da
We did all we could	최선을 다했습니다	chwe-son da-het-sup-nee-da

DISCHARGE

You have...(See Medical Prob List)	아래와 같은 증상 이 있습니다.	
He/she is going to stay in the hospital	입원 하실겁니다	ip-won ha-se-yo
Take "X" pills "Y" times a day for "Z" days	하루에 ____번 ____일 동안 복용 하세요	ha-roo ____ ge____ bun____eel dong-an bok-yong ha-se-yo
Pills	약	yak
Antibiotics	항생제	hang-seng-je
Before/after meals	식전 / 식후	shik-jun/ shik-hoo
Return to the ER if...	만일 ____경우 응급실로 다시 오 세요	____ung-gup-sheel ro da-shee o-se-yo
Follow up at "X" on "Y"	다음 진찰은 _____ 입니다	da-um jin-chal un _____ip-nee-da

You're welcome	천만에요	CHUN-man-e-yo
Goodbye	안녕히 가세요	an-NYUNG-hee ga-se-yo

MEDICAL PROBS

AIDS/HIV	에이즈 / 후천성 면역 결핍증	AIDS (e-ee-z)
Anemia	빈혈	been-hyul
Arrhythmia	부정맥	boo-jung-mek
Arthritis	관절	gwan-jul
Asthma	천식	chun-shik
Bronchitis	기관지염	gee-gan-jee-yom
Cancer	암	am
Cirrhosis	간경변	gan-gyong-byun
Cholesterol	콜레스트롤	kol-le-s-te-rol
Cold	감기	gam-gee
Constipation	변비	byon-bee
Cyst	낭종	nang-jong
Diabetes	당뇨	dang-nyo
Dialysis	투석	too-suk
Diverticulitis	게실염	ge-shee-ryom
Emphysema	기종	gee-jong
Fibroids	섬유종	sum-yoo-jong
Fracture	골절	gol-jul
Flu	독감	do-kam/gam-gee
Gallstones	담석	dam-suk
Gastritis/GERD	위염	wee-yum
Hepatitis	간염	gan-yum

(cont.)

Heart attack	심장 발작 / 심근경색	shim-jang bal-jak
Heart disease	심장병	shim-jang-byung
Heart failure	심장마비	shim-jang ma-bee
Hypertension	고혈압	go-hyu-rap
Indigestion	소화불량	so-hwa bool-yang
Kidney stone	신장 결석	shin-jang gyul-suk
Lupus	낭창 / 루푸스	nang-chang/ loo-poo-s
Migraine	편두통	pyun-doo-tong
Murmur	심장 잡음	shim-jang jab-um
Pacemaker	맥박 조정기	maek-bak jo-jung-gee
Pneumonia	폐렴	pe-ryum
Seizures	간질	gan-jeel
STD	성병	sung byung
Stroke	뇌졸중	nwe- jol-jung
Ulcer	궤양	gwe-yang
Ulcerative colitis	궤양성 대장염	de-jang-yum
UTI	요로 감염증	so-byon gam-yum-jung
BODY PARTS		
Abdomen	복부 / 배	ba-e
Ankle	발목	bal-mok
Appendix	맹장	meng-jang
Arm	팔	pal
Artery	동맥	dong-mek
Back	등	dung
Bladder	방광	bang-gwang
Blood	피	pee

Bone	뼈	pyo
Brain	뇌	n-we
Breast	유방	yoo-bang
Calf	종아리	jong-a-ree
Chest	가슴	ga-sum
Chin	턱	tuk
Ear	귀	g-wee
Elbow	팔꿈치	pal-koom-chee
Eye	눈	noon
Face	얼굴	ur-gool
Finger	손가락	son-ga-rak
Foot	발	bal
Hand	손	son
Head	머리	mu-ree
Heart	심장	shim-jang
Gallbladder	담낭	dam-nang
Jaw	턱	tuk
Joint	관절	gwan-jul
Kidney	신장	shin-jang
Knee	무릎	moo-rup
Leg	다리	da-ree
Liver	간	gan
Mouth	입	ip
Muscle	근육	g-nyook
Neck	목	mok
Nerve	신경	shin-gyung

(cont.)

Nose	코	ko
Ovary	난소	nan-so
Pancreas	췌장	chwe-jang
Penis	음경 / 페니스	pe-nee-s
Prostate	전립선	jun-rip-sun
Rectum	직장	jik-jang
Rib	갈비뼈	gal-bee
Shoulder	어깨	u-ke
Skin	피부	pee-boo
Spleen	비장	bee-jang
Spine	척추	chuk-choo
Stomach	배	bae
Teeth	치아	chee-a
Testicle	고환	go-hwan
Throat	인후 / 식도	SHIK-do
Thyroid	갑상선	gap-sang-sun
Toe	발가락	bal-ga-rak
Tonsils	편도선	pyon-do-sun
Tongue	혀	hyu
Uterus	자궁	ja-goong
Vagina	질	jeel
Vein	혈관	hyol-gwan
Wrist	손목	son-mok
NUMBERS		
How many (times)?	얼마만큼? / 몇번?	MYUT-bun?
0	공 / 제로	gong/je-ro
1	하나	hana

Korean—한국어

2	둘	dool
3	세	set
4	넷	net
5	다섯	da-sut
6	여섯	yu-sut
7	일곱	eel-gop
8	여덟	yo-dul
9	아홉	a-hop
10	열	yol
11	열 하나	yol-hana
20	이십	ee-ship
30	삼십	sam-ship
40	사십	sa-ship
50	오십	o-ship
60	육십	yook-ship
70	칠십	chil-ship
80	팔십	pal-ship
90	구십	goo-ship
100	백	bek

Mandarin Chinese—国语 (國語)

WORD/PHRASE	MANDARIN	PĪN YĪN	ENGLISH PRONUNCIATION
Mandarin Chinese	国语 (國語)	Guó yǔ	gwa ü
INTRODUCTION & REGISTRATION			
Hello	您好	Nín hǎo	neen hau
I am a doctor / nurse (add your name)	我是__医(醫)生/护(護)士	Wǒ shì (add your name) "yī shēng" (doctor) / "hù shi" (nurse)	wa shir (add your name) "ee shung" (doctor) / "hoo shir" (nurse)
What is your name?	名字?	Míng zi?	ming zu?
Who is your doctor?	您的医(醫)生是谁(誰)?	Nín de yī shēng shì shéi?	neen de ee shung shir shey?
How old are you?	几岁 (幾歲)?	Jǐ suì?	zhee swey?
Birthdate?	生日?	Shēng rì?	shung ri?
Telephone number?	电话号码 (電話號碼)?	Diàn huà hào mǎ?	dee-en hwa hau ma?
Address?	地址?	Dì zhǐ?	dee zhir?
Social security number?	社会(會)安全号码 (號碼)?	Shè huì ān quán hào mǎ?	shu hwe æn chyuen hau ma?
Insurance?	保险(險)?	Báo xiǎn?	bau shyen?
BASICS			
Do you understand?	懂吗(嗎)?	Dǒng ma?	dong ma?
Yes	是/有	Shì/Yǒu	shir/yo

(cont.)

No	不是/没有	Bú shì/Méi yǒu	boo shir/mey yo
Please	请(請)	Qǐng	cheeng
Thank you	谢谢(謝謝)	Xiè xie	shye shye
Sorry	对(對)不起	Duì bu qǐ	dwe boo chee
I don't understand	我不懂	Wǒ bù dǒng	wa boo dong
Repeat	再说(說)一次	Zài shuō yī cì	zay showa ee tsu
Speak slowly	慢慢说(說)	Màn màn shuō	mæn mæn showa
Answer "yes" or "no"	回答是或者不是	Huí dá shì huò zhě bú shì	hwe da shir hwa zhu boo shir
Here	这(這)里	Zhè lǐ	zhu lee
This	这个(這個)	Zhè ge	zhu gu
It's alright (consoling)	别担(擔)心	Bié dān xīn	bye dæn sheen
I'll be right back	我马(馬)上回来(來)	Wǒ mǎ shàng huí lái	wa ma shang hwe lay

GENERAL

What's wrong?	什么(麼)事?	Shén me shì?	shun mu shir?
Pain	痛	Tòng	tong
Do you have pain?	有没有痛?	Yǒu méi yǒu tòng?	yo mey yo tong?
Does the pain radiate?	痛蔓延马(馬)?	Tòng màn yán ma?	tong mæn yen ma?
Where (show me)	哪里(裡)?	Ná lǐ?	na lee?
Gone now	没有了	Méi yǒu le	mey yo lu
Still present	还(還)有	Hái yǒu	hay yo

Mandarin Chinese—国语 (國語)

Sudden/gradual onset	突然	Tū rán	too ræn
What bothers you the most?	什么(麼)最不舒服?	Shén me zuì bù shū fu?	shun mu zwe boo shoo foo?
Why did you come today?	您来(來)的原因是什么(麼)?	Nín lái de yuán yīn shì shén me?	neen lay du yu-wen een shir shun mu?
QUALITY			
If '0' is no pain and 10 is maximum pain, what number do you have now?	从(從)零到十,零不痛,十最痛,您现(現)在有多痛?	Cóng líng dào shí, líng bú tòng, shí zuì tòng, nín xiàn zài yǒu duō tòng?	tsong leeng dau shir, leeng boo tong, shir zwe tong, neen shee-en zay yo dowa tong?
Burning	烧(燒)的感觉(覺)	Shāo de gǎn jué	shau du gæn zhye
Constant	不停的	Bù tíng de	boo teeng du
Dull	不太感觉(覺)到的痛	Bú tài gǎn jué dào de tòng	boo tay gæn zhye dau du tong
Intermittent	断断续续(斷斷續續)	Duàn duàn xù xù	dwan dwan shü shü
Pressure	压(壓)迫的感觉(覺)	Yā pò de gǎn jué	ya pwa du gæn zhye
Severe	很痛	Hěn tòng	hen tong
Sharp/prickly pains	刺的感觉(覺)	Cì de gǎn jué	tsu du gæn zhye
Throbbing	跳动(動)的感觉(覺)	Tiào dòng de gǎn jué	tyeau dong du gæn zhye
ASSOCIATED SYMPTOMS			
Onset during… (before/after)	_的时(時)候开(開)始	_ de shí hòu kāi shǐ	_ du shir ho kay shir

(cont.)

Worse (with…)	__的时(時)候会变坏(會變壞)	__ de shí hòu huì biàn huài	__ du shir ho hwe bee-en hwe-ay
Better (with…)	__的时(時)候会变(會變)好	__ de shí hòu huì biàn hǎo	__ du shir ho hwe bee-en hau
Cough	咳嗽	Ké sòu	ku so
Deep breath	深呼吸	Shēn hū xī	shun hoo shee
Emotional upset	烦恼(煩惱)	Fán nǎo	fæn nau
Food	吃东(東)西	Chī dōng xi	chir dong shee
Movement	动(動)作	Dòng zuò	dong zwa
Nothing	没什么(麼)	Méi shén me	mey shun mu
Positioning	换姿势(换姿势)	Huàn zī shì	hwan zu shir
Rest	休息	Xiū xi	shyo shee
Walking	走路	Zǒu lù	zo loo
TIME COURSE			
For how long?	多久?	Duō jiǔ?	dowa zhyo?
Today	今天	Jīn tiān	zheen tyen
Yesterday	昨天	Zuó tiān	zwa tyen
How many…	多少…	Duō shǎo…	dowa shau…
Months/ weeks/days/ hours/ seconds	月/星期/日/小时(時)/秒	Yuè/xīng qī/ ri/xiǎo shí/ miǎo	yuwe/sheeng chee/ ir/shee-yaau shir/ mee-au
Still present?	还(還)有吗(嗎)?	Hái yǒu ma?	hay yo ma?
Gone now?	没了吗(嗎)?	Méi le ma?	mey lu ma?
How long did it last? (See Numbers List)	有了多久?	Yǒu le duō jiǔ?	yo lu dowa zheeyo

Have you had this before?	以前有过吗(過嗎)?	Yǐ qián yǒu guò ma?	ee chyen yo gwa ma?
How many times?	几(幾)次?	Jǐ cì?	zhee tsu?
When was the last time?	上次是什么时(麼時)候?	Shàng cì shì shén me shí hòu?	shang tsu shir shun mu shir ho?
New	新	Xīn	sheen
Old	旧(舊)	Jiù	zhyo
CONTEXT			
Did you...?	有没有...?	Yǒu méi yǒu...?	yo mey yo ...?
fall	摔倒	Shuāi dǎo	shwaay dau
trip	绊(絆)倒	Bàn dǎo	bæn dau
faint	昏倒	Hūn dǎo	hwen dau
twist	扭到	Niǔ dào	nyo dau
get hit	被撞到	Bèi zhuàng dào	bey zhwang dau
get burned	被烧(燒)到	Bèi shāo dào	bey shau dau
get assaulted	被打到	Bèi dǎ dào	bey da dau
get bitten (human/dog/cat/insect)	被咬到	Bèi yǎo dào	bey yeau dau
PAST MEDICAL HISTORY			
Take medication?	您有吃药吗(藥嗎)?	Nín yǒu chī yào ma?	neen yo chir yeau ma?
(aspirin/antibiotics)	阿斯匹林/抗生素	Ā sī pǐ lín/kàng shēng sù	a see pee leen/kang shung soo

(cont.)

Do you have (See also Medical Problem List)…	您有没有...?	Nín yǒu méi yǒu...?	neen yo mey yo...?
allergies	过敏(過敏)	Guò mǐn	gwa meen
medical problems	什么(麼)病	Shén me bìng	shun mu beeng
Do you have problems of the…(see Body Parts List)	您有没有__的问题(問題)	Nín yǒu méi yǒu__ de wèn tí	neen yo mey yo__ du wen tee
SURGICAL HISTORY			
Have you had surgery?	动过(動過)手术吗(術嗎)?	Dòng guò shǒu shù ma?	dong gwa sho shoo ma?
Surgery on/"to remove"…(see Body Parts List)	__动过(動過)手术(術)	__ dòng guò shǒu shù	__ dong gwa sho shoo
SOCIAL HISTORY			
Smoke?	抽烟吗(抽煙嗎)?	Chōu yān ma?	cho yan ma?
Drink?	喝酒吗(嗎)?	Hē jiǔ ma?	hu zheeo ma?
Take drugs?	用毒品吗(嗎)?	Yòng dú pǐn ma?	yong doo peen ma?
Recent travel?	最近旅行吗(嗎)?	Zuì jìn lǚ xíng ma?	zwe zheen lü sheeng ma?
Are you sexually active?	您有性行为吗(為嗎)?	Nín yǒu xìng xíng wéi ma?	neen yo sheeng sheeng we ma?
Do you use condoms?	您用保险(險)套吗(嗎)?	Nín yòng bǎo xiǎn tào ma?	neen yo bau shen tau ma?
Homosexual	同性恋(戀)	Tóng xìng liàn	tong sheeng lee-en

Mandarin Chinese—国语 (國語)

SYSTEMS REVIEW			
Do you have...	您有__吗(嗎)?	Nín yǒu __ ma?	neen yo __ ma?
GENERAL			
Fever	发烧(發燒)	Fā shāo	fa shau
Chills	寒颤(顫)	Hán chàn	hæn chæn
Weight loss	瘦了	Shòu le	sho lu
Fatigue	疲劳(勞)	Pí láo	pee lau
Sick contact	跟病人接触(觸)	Gēn bìng rén jiē chù	gun beeng run zhe choo
HEENT			
Sore throat	喉咙(嚨)痛	Hóu lóng tòng	ho long tong
Runny nose	流鼻涕	Liú bí tì	leeo bee tee
Nosebleed	鼻血	Bí xuě	bee shwe
Ear pain	耳中疼痛	Ěr zhòng téng tòng	ar zhong tung tong
Ear ringing	耳鸣(鳴)	Ěr míng	ar meeng
Decreased hearing	听觉减落(聽覺減落)	Tīng jué jiǎn luò	teeng zhwee zhee-en lwa
EYE			
Eye pain	眼睛痛	Yǎn jīng tòng	yen zheeng tong
Blurry vision	视线(視線)模糊	Shì xiàn mó hú	shir shee-en mwa hoo
Diplopia	重影	Chóng yǐng	chong eeng
Foreign body sensation	眼睛有东(東)西的感觉(覺)	Yǎn jīng yǒu dōng xi de gǎn jué	yen zheeng yo dong shee du gæn zhwe
Contact lenses	隐(隱)形眼镜(鏡)	Yǐn xíng yǎn jìng	een sheeng yen zheeng

(cont.)

CARDIAC			
Chest pain	胸痛	Xiōng tòng	sheeong tong
Palpitations	心悸	Xīn jì	sheen zhee
Orthopnea	躺下来的时(時)候感到喘不过气(過氣)	Tǎng xià lái de shí hòu gǎn dào chuǎn bú guò qì	tang shee-a lay du shir ho gæn dau chwa-æn boo gwa chee
Dyspnea on exertion	用力的时(時)候感到喘不过气(過氣)	Yòng lì de shí hòu gǎn dào chuǎn bú guò qì	yong lee du shir ho gæn dau chwa-æn boo gwa chee
Fainting (syncope)	昏倒	Hūn dào	hwen dau
Leg swelling	腿有水肿(腫)	Tuǐ yǒu shuǐ zhǒng	twe yo shwe zhong
How many pillows?	几个(幾個)枕头(頭)	Jǐ ge zhěn tóu	zhee gu zhen to
PULMONARY			
Trouble breathing	呼吸困难(難)	Hū xī kùn nán	hoo shee kwen næn
SOB	喘不过气(過氣)	Chuǎn bú guò qì	chwæn boo gwa chee
Cough	咳嗽	Ké sòu	ku so
Sputum	痰	Tán	tæn
Pain on inspiration	呼吸的时候痛(時候痛)	Hū xī de shí hòu tòng	hoo shee du shir ho tong
Hemoptysis	咯血	Ké xuě	ku shwe
GI			
Abdominal pain	腹痛	Fù tòng	foo tong
Nausea	恶(惡)心	Ě xīn	u sheen
Vomiting	吐	Tù	too

Vomiting blood	吐血	Tù xuě	too shwe
Coffee ground emesis	吐血块(塊)	Tù xuě kuài	too shwe kwaay
Anorexia	厌(厭)食	Yàn shí	yen shir
Diarrhea	腹泻(瀉)	Fù xiè	foo shee-e
Difficulty swallowing	吞咽困难(難)	Tūn yàn kùn nán	twen yen kwen næn
BRBPR	粪(糞)便有血	Fèn biàn yóu xuě	fen bee-en yo shwe
Melena	黑便	Hē biàn	hey bee-en
Pain after eating	吃饭(飯)以后(後)胃痛	Chī fàn yǐ hòu wèi tòng	chir fæn ee ho we tong
Worms	寄生虫(蟲)	Jì shēng chóng	zhee shung chong
Constipation	便秘	Biàn mì	bee-en mee
GU			
Painful urination	小便时候痛(時候痛)	Xiǎo biàn shí hòu tòng	shee-au bee-en shir ho tong
Urgent urination	小便有忍不住的感觉(覺)	Xiǎo biàn yǒu rěn bu zhù de gǎn jué	shee-au bee-en yo run boo zhoo du gæn zhwe
Frequent urination	小便比平时(時)多	Xiǎo biàn bǐ píng shí duō	shee-au bee-en bee peeng shir dwa
Bloody urination	小便有血	Xiǎo biàn yóu xuě	shee-au bee-en yo shwe
Discharge: vaginal/ penile	"阴(陰)道"/"阴茎(陰莖)"有分泌物	"Yīn dào"/"yīn jīng" yǒu fēn mì wù	"een dau"/"een zheeng" yo fun mee woo
PSYCH			
Anxiety	紧张(緊張)	Jǐn zhāng	zheen zhang

(cont.)

Depression	忧郁(憂鬱)	Yōu yù	yo ü
Suicidal thoughts	自杀(殺)想法	Zì shā xiáng fǎ	zu sha shee-ang fa
Homicidal thoughts	伤(傷)人想法	Shāng rén xiáng fǎ	shang run shee-ang fa
Medication overdose	用药过(藥過)多	Yòng yào guò duō	yong yeau go-wa do-wa
Hear voices	幻觉(覺)	Huàn jué	hwan zhwe
NEURO			
Headache	头(頭)痛	Tóu tòng	to tong
Worst headache of life	头从来(頭從來)没有那么(麼)痛过(過)	Tóu cóng lái méi yǒu nà me tòng guò	to tsong lay mey yo na mu tong go-wa
Weakness	弱	Ruò	rowa
Dizzy	昏	Hūn	hwen
What is your name?	名字?	Míng zi?	ming zu?
Where are we?	我们(們)在哪里(裡)?	Wǒ mén zài ná lǐ?	wa mun zay na lee?
What is the year/month/date?	哪一年/几(幾)月/几号(幾號)?	Nǎ yì nián/jǐ yuè/jǐ hào?	na yee nee-en/zhee yewe/zhee hau?
Bowel dysfunction	胃肠(腸)不正常	Wèi cháng bú zhèng cháng	we chang boo zhung chang
Bladder dysfunction	膀胱不正常	Páng guāng bú zhèng cháng	pang gwang boo zhung chang
Photophobia	畏光	Wèi guāng	we gwang
Tingling/numbness	麻	Má	ma
Decreased strength in... (See Body Parts List)	__无(無)力吗(嗎)?	__ wú lì ma?	__ woo lee ma?

Seizure	癫痫(癲癇)	Diān xián	dee-en shee-en
Difficulty walking	走路有困难(難)	Zǒu lù yǒu kùn nán	zo loo yo kwen næn
Difficulty speaking	说话(說話)有困难(難)	Shuō huà yǒu kùn nán	showa hwa yo kwen næn
Spinning (vertigo)	头(頭)昏	Tóu hūn	to hwen
Confusion	迷乱(亂)	Mí luàn	mee l-weæn
MISC			
Lump	肿块(腫塊)	Zhǒng kuài	zhong kwaay
Itching	痒(癢)	Yǎng	yang
Bruising	淤血	Yū xuě	Ü shwe
Rash	发(發)疹	Fā zhěn	fa zhen
Swelling	肿胀(脹)	Zhǒng zhàng	zhong zhang
Jaundice (yellow skin)	疸	Dǎn	dæn
GYNECOLOGIC			
Vaginal bleeding	阴(陰)道出血	Yīn dào chū xuě	een dau choo shwe
Heavy	量多	Liàng duō	leeang dowa
Irregular	不规则(規則)	Bu4 guī zé	boo gwe zu
Absent	没有	Méi yǒu	mey yo
Vaginal discharge	阴(陰)道有分泌物	Yīn dào yǒu fēn mì wù	een dau yo fun mee woo
Pelvic pain	骨盆痛	Gǔ pén tòng	goo pun tong
Rape	强奸(強姦)	Qiáng jiān	chee-ang zhee-en
Pain with intercourse	性交的(時)候有痛	Xìng jiāo de shí hòu yǒu tòng	sheeng zhee-au du shir ho yo tong
Contraceptive	避孕	Bì yùn	bee ün

(cont.)

Mandarin Chinese—国语 (國語)

OBSTETRIC			
Are you pregnant?	您有怀(懷)孕吗(嗎)?	Nín yǒu huái yùn ma?	neen yo hwaay ün ma?
LMP how many days ago?	上次月经(經)是什么时(麼時)候?	Shàng cì yuè jīng shì shén me shí hòu?	shang tsu yue zheeng shir shen mu shir ho?
Times pregnant?	怀(懷)孕过几(過幾)次?	Huái yùn guò jǐ cì?	hwaay ün gwa zhee tsu?
Times delivered?	生产过几(產過幾)次?	Shēng chǎn guò jǐ cì?	sheng chæn gwa zhee tsu?
Miscarriage	流产(產)	Liú chǎn	leeo chæn
Abortion	堕胎	Duò tāi	dwa tay
Fluid leakage	羊水流出	Yáng shuǐ liú chū	yang shwe leeo choo
Contraction	阵(陣)痛	Zhèn tòng	zhen tong
Fetal movement	胎动(動)	Tāi dòng	tay dong

TRAUMA			
How many hours ago did you eat last?	上次吃东(東)西是几个(幾個)小时(時)以前?	Shàng cì chī dōng xi shì jǐ gè xiǎo shí yǐ qián?	shang tsu chir dong shee shir zhee gu sheeau shir ee chee-en?
Lost consciousness?	失去知觉吗(覺嗎)?	Shī qù zhī jué ma?	shir chū zhir zhwe ma?
Tetanus within 5 years?	五年之内(內)有打过(過)破伤风预(傷風預)防针吗(針嗎)?	Wǔ nián zhī nèi yǒu dǎ guò pò shāng fēng yù fáng zhēn ma?	woo nee-en zhir ney yo da gwa pwa shang fong ü fang zhun ma?

PEDIATRIC			
How old?	几岁(幾歲)?	Jǐ suì?	zhee swe?
Vaccines up to date?	预(預)防针(針)打全了吗(嗎)?	Yù fáng zhēn dǎ quán le ma?	Ü fang zhun da chwen lu ma?

Urinating normally	小便正常吗(嗎)?	Xiǎo biàn zhèng cháng ma?	shee-au bee-en zhung chang ma?
Taking liquids	喝东(東)西	Hē dōng xi	hu dong shee
Increased crying	比平常哭得多	Bǐ píng cháng kū de duō	bee peeng chang koo du dowa
Ingestion	摄(攝)食	Shè shí	shu shir
Foreign body	异(異)物	Yì wù	ee woo
Premature	早产(產)	Záo chǎn	zau chæn
Birth complications	生产并发(產併發)症	Shēng chǎn bìng fā zhèng	shung chæn beeng fa zhung
PHYSICAL EXAM/INSTRUCTION			
Sit down (please)	请(請)坐下	Qǐng zuò xià	cheeng zwa sheea
Lie down	躺下	Tǎng xià	tang sheea
Come here	过来(過來)	Guò lái	gwa lay
Relax	放松(鬆)	Fàng sōng	fang song
Don't move	不要动(動)	Bú yào dòng	boo yau dong
Open your mouth	嘴巴张开(張開)	Zuǐ ba zhāng kāi	zwe ba zhang kay
Say "ahh"	说(說)"ahh"	Shuō "ahh"	showa "ahh"
Swallow	吞一下	Tūn yī xià	twen ee sheea
Breath deeply	深呼吸	Shēn hū xī	shun hoo shee
Hold your breath	憋住气(氣)	Biē zhù qì	bee-e zhoo chee
Cough	咳嗽	Ké sòu	ku so
Push	推	Tuī	twe
Pull	拉	Lā	la

(cont.)

Follow my finger	眼睛跟著我的手指	Yǎn jīng gēn zhe wǒ de shóu zhī	yen zheeng gen zhu wa de sho zhir
Close your eyes	眼睛闭(閉)著	Yǎn jīng bì zhe	yen zheeng bee zhu
Smile	笑	Xiào	sheeau
Can you feel this?	感觉(覺)到吗(嗎)?	Gǎn jué dào ma?	gæn zhwe dau ma?
Copy this (movement)	跟著我做	Gēn zhe wǒ zuò	gen zhu wa zwa
I am going to put a finger in your rectum	我要把手指放在您的肛门里(門裡)面	Wǒ yào bǎ shóu zhī fàng zài nín de gāng mén lǐ miàn	wa yau ba sho zhir fang zay neen du gang mun lee mee-en
I am going to examine your vagina	我要作阴(陰)道检(檢)查	Wǒ yào zuò yīn dào jiǎn chá	wa yau zwa een dau zhee-en cha
REASSESSMENT			
Do you feel better?	有没有舒服一点(點)	Yǒu méi yǒu shū fu yī diǎn?	yo mey yo shoo foo ee dee-en?
Do you feel worse?	有没有更不舒服	Yǒu méi yǒu gèng bù shū fu?	yo mey yo gung boo shoo foo?
PATIENT WORDS			
I hurt	痛	Tòng	tong
Help!	救命	Jiù mìng!	zhee-o meeng!
Bathroom	厕所(廁所)	Cè suǒ	tsu swa
Food	食物	Shí wù	shir woo
Water	水	Shuǐ	shwe
PROCEDURES & CONSENT			
You need...	您需要…	Nín xū yào...	neen shü yau...

Injection	打针(針)	Dǎ zhēn	da zhen
Stiches	缝(縫)合	Féng hé	fung hu
Cast	石膏	Shí gāo	shir gau
Crutches	拐杖	Guǎi zhàng	gwaay zhang
Perform surgery on the... (See Body Parts List)	要动(動)__手术(術)	Yào dòng __ shǒu shù	yau dong __ sho shoo
The risks are...	有一些风险(風險)是…	Yǒu yī xiē fēng xiǎn shì…	yo yee shee-e fung shee-en shir…
Bleeding	流血	Liú xuě	leeo shwe
Infection	感染	Gán rǎn	gæn ræn
Scar	疤痕	Bā hén	ba hen
Repeat procedure	重做	Chóng zuò	chong zwa
Iodine	碘	Diǎn	dee-en
Damage to your...(See Body Parts List)	有受伤(傷)	__ yǒu shòu shāng	__ yo sho shang
Sign here	这里签(這裡簽)名	Zhè lǐ qiān míng	zhu lee chee-en meeng
TESTS			
X-ray	"X"光检(檢)查	"X" guāng jiǎn chá	"x" gwang zhee-en cha
C.A.T. Scan	电脑扫(電腦掃)描	Diàn nǎo sǎo miáo	dee-en nau sau meeau
Ultrasound	超音波检(檢)查	Chāo yīn bō jiǎn chá	chau yeen bwa zhee-en cha

(cont.)

Catheterization/bladder catheter	插管/导(導)尿管	Chā guǎn/dǎo niào guǎn	cha gwan/dau nee-au gwan
Colonoscopy (from below)/Endoscopy (from above)	大肠镜(腸鏡)	Dà cháng jìng	da chang zheeng
Endoscopy	内窥镜检(内窺鏡檢)查	Nèi kuī jìng jiǎn chá	ney kwe zheeng zhee-en cha
END OF LIFE			
Do you want us to…	您要不要我们(們)…	Nín yào bú yào wǒ mén…	neen yau boo yau wa mun…
Perform CPR	您要不要我们(們)作心肺复苏术(復甦術)	Zuò xīn fèi fù sū shù	zwa sheen fey foo soo shoo
Defibrillate	电击(電擊)	Diàn jī	dee-en zhee
Intubate	插管	Chā guǎn	cha gwan
He/she is dead	他/她去世了	Tā qù shì le	ta chü shir lu
We did all we could	我们(們)尽力了	Wǒ mén jìn lì le	wa mun zheen lee lu
DISCHARGE			
You have… (See Medical Prob List)	您有…	Nín yǒu…	neen yo…
He/she is going to stay in the hospital	他/她需要留在医(醫)院	Tā xū yào liú zài yī yuàn	ta shü yau lee-o zay yee yuwen
Take "X" pills "Y" times a day for "Z" days	一次吃__粒. 每天吃__次, 这样(這樣)下去__天.	Yī cì chī "X" lì. Měi tiān chī "Y" cì. Zhè yàng xià qù "Z" tiān.	ee tsi chir "X" lee. mey tee-en chir "Y" tsi. zhu yang sheea chü Z" tee-en.
Pills	药(藥)丸	Yào wán	yau wan

Mandarin Chinese—国语(國語)

Antibiotics	抗生素	Kàng shēng sù	kang shung soo
Before/after meals	吃饭(飯)之前/后(後)	Chī fàn zhī qián/hòu	chir fæn zhir chee-en/ho
Return to the ER if…	如果__回急诊(診)室	Rú guǒ __ huí jí zhěn shì	roo gwa __ hwe zhee zhun shir
Follow up at "X" on "Y"	__月__号(號)需要回__检(檢)查	"Y" (month) yuè "Y" (date) hào xū yào huí "X" (place) jiǎn chá	"Y" (month) yewe "Y" (date) hau shü yau hwe "X" (place) zhee-en cha
You're welcome	不客气(氣)	Bú kè qi	boo ku chee
Goodbye	再见(見)	Zài jiàn	zay zhee-en
MEDICAL PROBS			
AIDS/HIV	艾滋病/艾滋病毒	Ài zī bìng/Ài zī bìng dú	ay zu beeng/ay zu beeng doo
Anemia	贫(貧)血	Pín xuě	peen shwe
Arrhythmia	心律失调(調)	Xīn lǜ shī tiáo	sheen lü shir teeau
Arthritis	关节(關節)炎	Guān jié yán	gwaæn zhee-e yen
Asthma	气(氣)喘	Qì chuǎn	chee chwan
Bronchitis	支气(氣)管炎	Zhī qì guǎn yán	zhir chee gwaæn yen
Cancer	癌症	Ái Zhèng	ay zhung
Cirrosis	肝硬化	Gān yìng huà	gæn eeng hwaay
Cholesterol	胆(膽)固醇	Dǎn gù chún	dæn goo chwen
Cold	感冒	Gǎn mào	gæn mau
Constipation	便秘	Biàn mì	bee-en mee
Cyst	囊肿(腫)	Náng zhǒng	nang zhong

(cont.)

Diabetes	糖尿病	Táng niào bìng	tang nee-au beeng
Dialysis	血液透析	Xuè yè tòu xī	shwe ye to shee
Diverticulitis	憩室炎	Qì shì yán	chee shir yen
Emphysema	肺气肿(氣腫)	Fèi qì zhǒng	fey chee zhong
Fibroids	纤维(纖維)瘤	Xiān wéi liú	shee-en we leeo
Fracture	骨折	Gǔ zhé	goo zhu
Flu	流感	Liú gǎn	leeo gæn
Gallstones	胆(膽)石	Dǎn shí	dæn shir
Gastritis/GERD	胃炎/胃灼热(熱)	Wèi yán/Wèi zhuó rè	we yen/we zhwa ru
Hepatitis	肝炎	Gān yán	gæn yen
Heart attack	心脏(臟)病发(發)作	Xīn zàng bìng fā zuò	sheen zang beeng fa zwa
Heart disease	心脏(臟)病	Xīn zàng bìng	sheen zang beeng
Heart failure	心脏(臟)衰竭	Xīn zàng shuāi jié	sheen zang shwaay zhee-e
Hypertension	高血压(壓)	Gāo xuě yā	gau shwe ya
Indigestion	消化不良	Xiāo huà bù liáng	shee-au hwa boo leeang
Kidney stone	肾结(腎結)石	Shèn jié shí	shun zhee-e shir
Lupus	狼疮(瘡)	Láng chuāng	lang chwang
Migraine	偏头(頭)痛	Piān tóu tòng	pee-en to tong
Murmur	心脏杂(臟雜)音	Xīn zàng zá yīn	sheen zang za yeen
Pacemaker	心电起博(電起博)器	Xīn diàn qǐ bó qì	sheen dee-en chee bwa chee
Pneumonia	肺炎	Fèi yán	fey yen
Seizures	癫痫(癲癇)	Diān xián	dee-en shee-en

Mandarin Chinese—国语 (國語)

STD	性病	Xìng bìng	sheeng beeng
Stroke	中风(風)	Zhòng fēng	zhong fung
Ulcer	溃疡(潰瘍)	Kuì yáng	kwe yang
Ulcerative colitis	溃疡(潰瘍)性大肠(腸)炎	Kuì yáng xìng dà cháng yán	kwe yang sheeng da chang yen
UTI	尿道感染	Niào dào gán rǎn	neeau dau gæn ran
BODY PARTS			
Abdomen	肚子	Dù zi	doo zu
Ankle	脚(腳)踝	Jiǎo huái	zheeau hooay
Appendix	盲肠(腸)	Máng cháng	mang chang
Arm	手臂	Shǒu bèi	sho bey
Artery	动脉(動脈)	Dòng mài	dong may
Back	背部	Bèi bù	bey boo
Bladder	膀胱	Páng guāng	pang gwang
Blood	血	Xuě	shwe
Bone	骨骼	Gǔ gé	goo gu
Brain	脑(腦)子	Nǎo zi	nau zu
Breast	乳房	Rǔ fáng	roo fang
Calf	小腿	Xiáo tuǐ	shee-au tooey
Chest	胸部	Xiōng bù	shee-ong boo
Chin	下巴	Xià ba	shee-a ba
Ear	耳朵	Ěr duō	ar dowa
Elbow	肘	Zhǒu	zho
Eye	眼睛	Yǎn jīng	yen zheeng
Face	脸(臉)	Liǎn	lee-en
Finger	手指	Shóu zhī	sho zhir

(cont.)

Foot	脚(脚)	Jiǎo	zhee-au
Hand	手	Shǒu	sho
Head	头(頭)	Tóu	to
Heart	心脏(臟)	Xīn zàng	sheen zang
Gallbladder	胆(膽)囊	Dǎn náng	dæn nang
Jaw	颚(顎)	È	u
Joint	关节(關節)	Guān jié	gwan zhee-e
Kidney	(腎)	Shèn	shen
Knee	膝盖(蓋)	Xī gài	shee gay
Leg	腿	Tuǐ	tooey
Liver	肝	Gān	gæn
Mouth	口	Kǒu	ko
Muscle	肌肉	Jī ròu	zhee ro
Neck	脖子	Bó zi	bwa zu
Nerve	神经(經)	Shén jīng	shen zheeng
Nose	鼻子	Bí zi	bee zu
Ovary	卵巢	Luǎn cháo	l-waæn chau
Pancreas	胰脏(臟)	Yí zàng	yee zang
Penis	阴茎(陰莖)	Yīn jīng	yeeng zheeng
Prostate	前列腺	Qián liè qiàn	chee-en lee-e chee-en
Rectum	直肠(腸)	Zhí cháng	zhir chang
Rib	肋骨	Lè gǔ	lu goo
Shoulder	肩膀	Jiān bǎng	zhee-en bang
Skin	皮肤(膚)	Pí fū	pee foo
Spleen	脾脏(臟)	Pí zàng	pee zang
Spine	脊椎骨	Jí zhuī gǔ	zhee zhwe goo

Stomach	胃	Wèi	we
Teeth	牙齿(齒)	Yá chǐ	ya chir
Testicle	睾丸	Gāo wán	gau wæn
Throat	喉咙(嚨)	Hóu lóng	ho long
Thyroid	甲狀腺	Jiǎ zhuàng xiàn	zhee-a zhooang shee-en
Toe	脚(腳)趾	Jiáo zhǐ	zhee-au zhir
Tonsils	扁桃体(體)	Biǎn táo tǐ	bee-en tau tee
Tongue	舌头(頭)	Shé tóu	shu to
Uterus	子宫(宮)	Zǐ gōng	zu gong
Vagina	阴(陰)道	Yīn dào	een dau
Vein	静脉(静脈)	Jìng mài	zheeng may
Wrist	手腕	Shǒu wàn	sho wæn

NUMBERS

How many (times)?	多少次?	Duō shǎo cì?	do-wa shau tsu?
0	零	Líng	leeng
1	一	Yī	ee
2	二	Èr	ar
3	三	Sān	sæn
4	四	Sì	su
5	五	Wǔ	oo
6	六	Liù	leeo
7	七	Qī	chee
8	八	Bā	ba
9	九	Jiǔ	zheeo
10	十	Shí	shir
11	十一	Shí yī	shir ee

20	二十	Èr shí	ar shir
30	三十	Sān shí	sæn shir
40	四十	Sì shí	su shir
50	五十	Wǔ shí	oo shir
60	六十	Liù shí	leeo shir
70	七十	Qī shí	chee shir
80	八十	Bā shí	ba shir
90	九十	Jiǔ shí	zheeo shir
100	一百	Yī bǎi	ee bay

Polish—Polski

WORD/ PHRASE	TRANSLATION	ENGLISH PRONUNCIATION
Polish	Polski	POL-skee
INTRODUCTION & REGISTRATION		
Hello	Dźień dobry	JEN DO-bri
I am a doctor / nurse *(add your name)*	Jestem Doktorem / pielęgniarką *(add your name)*	YES-tem dok-TOR-em / p-ye-leng-N-YAR-kang *(add your name)*
What is your name?	Jak się nazywasz?	yak sheng na-zi-VASH?
Who is your doctor?	Kto jest twoim doktorem?	k-TO yest t-VOY-eem dok-TOR-em?
How old are you?	Ile masz lat?	EE-le mash lat?
Birthdate?	Data urodzenia?	DA-ta oo-ro-JE-nee-ya?
Telephone number?	Numer telefonu?	NOO-mer te-LE-fo-noo?
Address?	Adres?	a-DRES?
Social security number?	Numer socjalnej bezpieczności	NOO-mer sots-YAL-ney bez-p-YECH-nosh-chee
Insurance?	Ubezpieczenie	oo-bez-p-ye-CHE-nee-ye
BASICS		
Do you understand?	Rozumiesz?	ro-zoo-MEE-yesh?
Yes	Tak	tak
No	Nie	n-YE
Please	Proszę	PRO-sheng

(cont.)

Thank you	Dziękuję	je*ng*-KOO-ye*ng*
Sorry	Przepraszam	p-she-PRA-sham
I don't understand	Nie rozumiem	n-YE ro-zoo-MEE-yem
Repeat	Powtórz	pov-TOOR-z
Speak slowly	Mów wolniej	MOOV VOL-nee-yey
Answer "yes" or "no"	Odpowiedz "tak" lub "nie"	od-PO-veej TAK loob n-YE
Here	Tutaj	TOO-tay
This	To	to
It's alright (consoling)	Nie martw się	n-ye MART-v she*ng*
I'll be right back	Zaraz wrócę	ZA-raz v-ROO-tse*ng*
GENERAL		
What's wrong?	Co dolega? / Co boli?	tso do-LE-ga/ tso bo-LEE ?
Pain	Ból	bool
Do you have pain?	Czy coś boli?	chi tsosh bo-LEE?
Does the pain radiate?	Czy ból promieniuje?	chi bool pro-m-ye-n-YOO-ye ?
Where (show me)	Gdzie? (pokaż)	g-JE? (po-KAZH)
Gone now	Już nie	yoozh n-YE?
Still present	Jeszcze istnieje	YESH-che eest-n-YE-ye
Sudden/gradual onset	nagłe / stopniowe najście	NAG-we / stop-n-YO-ve naysh-che
What bothers you the most?	Co dręczy cię najbardziej?	tso DRE*ng*-chi tse*ng* nay-BAR-jey?

Why did you come today?	Dlaczego przyszedłeś dzisiaj? (to a man); Dlaczego przyszedłaś dzisiaj? (to a woman)	d-la-CHE-go p-shi-SHED-wesh JEE-shay? (to a man); dla-CHE-go p-shi-SHED-wash JEE-shay? (to a woman)
QUALITY		
If '0' is no pain and 10 is maximum pain, what number do you have now?	Skala bólu jest od zero do dziesięciu, która liczba wskazuje twój ból?	SKA-la BOO-loo yest od ZE-ro do je-SHEng-soo k-TOOR-a LEECH-ba v-ska-ZOO-ye t-VOY bool
Burning	Palący	pa-LAng-tsi
Constant	Stały	STA-wi
Dull	Słaby	SWA-by
Intermittent	Sporadyczny	spor-a-DICH-ni
Pressure	Ciśnienie	chish-n-YE-n-ye
Severe	Mocny	MOTS-ni
Sharp/prickly pains	Ostre bóle	OS-tre BOO-le
Throbbing	Rwany	r-VA-ne
ASSOCIATED SYMPTOMS		
Onset during… (before/after)	Najście podczas (przed / po)	NAY-sh-che pod-CHAS (p-zhed / po)
Worse (with…)	Gorszy (z…)	GOR-shi (z…)
Better (with…)	Lepiej (z…)	L-YEP-yey (z…)
Cough	Kaszel	KA-shel
Deep breath	Głęboki oddech	gleng-BO-ki OD-dekh
Emotional upset	Rozterka psychiczna	roz-TER-ka p-si-KHEECH-na
Food	Żywność	zhiv-NOSH-ch

(cont.)

188 Polish—Polski

Movement	Ruch	rookh
Nothing	Nic	neets
Positioning	Pozycja	po-ZITS-ya
Rest	Odpoczynek	od-po-CHI-nek
Walking	Khodzenie / spacer	kho-JE-nee-ye / SPA-tser
TIME COURSE		
For how long?	Na jak długo?	na yak d-WOO-go
Today	Dzisiaj	JEE-shay
Yesterday	Wczoraj	v-chor-AY
How many...	Ile?	EE-le
Months/weeks/days/hours/seconds	miesiące / tygodnie /dni / godziny / sekundy	m-YE-sha*n*g-s / ti-GOD-n-ye / d-NEE / GO-jee-ni / se-KOON-di
Still present?	Jeszcze istnieje?	YESH-che eest-N-YE-ye?
Gone now?	Już nie?	yoozh n-YE?
How long did it last? (See Number List)	Jak długo to trwało?	yak d-WOO-go to tr-VA-wo?
Have you had this before?	Miałeś to wcześniej?	mee-YA-wesh to v-CHESH-n-yey?
How many times?	Ile razy?	EE-le ra-ZI?
When was the last time?	Kiedy tak było ostatni raz?	k-YE-di TAK BI-wo os-TAT-nee raz?
New	NOWY	NO-vi
Old	Stary	STA-ri
CONTEXT		
Did you...?	Czy...?	chi...?

Polish—Polski

fall	upadłeś (to a man); upadłaś (to a woman)	oo-PAD-wesh (to a man); oo-PAD-wash (to a woman)
trip	potknąłeś się (to a man); potknąłaś się (to a woman)	pot-K-NAng-wesh SHEng (to a man); pot-K-NAng-wash SHEng (to a woman)
faint	zemdlałeś (to a man); zemdlałaś (to a woman)	zemd-LA-wesh (to a man); zemd-LA-wash (to a woman)
twist	zwichnołeś (to a man); zwichnołaś (to a woman)	z-veekh-NO-wesh (to a man); z-veekh-NO-wash (to a woman)
get hit	byłeś uderzony (to a man); byłaś uderzona (to a woman)	BI-wesh oo-DER-zo-ni (to a man); BI-wash oo-DER-zo-na (to a woman)
get burned	byłeś poparzony (to a man); byłaś poparzona (to a woman)	BI-wesh po-PAR-zo-ni (to a man); BI-wash po-PAR-zo-na (to a woman)
get assaulted	zostałeś napadnięty (to a man); zostałaś napadnięta (to a woman)	zo-STA-wesh na-pad-NYEng-ti (to a man); zo-STA-wash na-pad-NYEng-ti (to a woman)
get bitten (human/dog/cat/insect)	byłeś podgryziony (to a man); byłaś podgryziona (to a woman)	BI-wesh pod-gri-ZYO-ni (to a man); BI-wash pod-gri-ZYO-na (to a woman)
PAST MEDICAL HISTORY		
Take medication?	Bierzesz lekarstwo?	b-YE-shesh le-KAR-st-vo?
(aspirin/antibiotics)	aspiryna / antybiotyki	as-pee-RI-na / an-ti-bee-O-ti-ki

(cont.)

Do you have (See also Medical Problem List)...	Czy masz...?	chi mash..?
allergies	alergię	a-LER-gee-ye*ng*
medical problems	Problemy medyczne	prob-LE-mi me-DICH-ne
Do you have problems of the...(see Body Parts List)	problemy z...	prob-LE-mi z...
SURGICAL HISTORY		
Have you had surgery?	Czy miałeś operacje? (to a man); Czy miałaś operacje? (to a woman)	chi mee-YA-wesh o-pe-RA-tsee-ye? (to a man); chi mee-YA-wash o-pe-RA-tsee-ye? (to a woman)
Surgery on/"to remove"...(see Body Parts List)	Operacje na...	o-PE-RA-tsee-ye na...
SOCIAL HISTORY		
Smoke?	Palisz papierosy?	PA-leesh pa-pee-RO-si?
Drink?	Pijesz alcohol?	PEE-yesh AL-ko-hol?
Take drugs?	Czy bierzesz narkotyki?	chi b-YE-zhesh nar-KO-ti-ki?
Recent travel?	Podróżowałeś ostatnio? (to a man); Podróżowałaś ostatnio? (to a woman)	pod-roo-zho-VA-wesh o-STAT-n-yo? (to a man); pod-roo-zho-VA-wash o-STAT-n-yo? (to a woman)
Are you sexually active?	Jesteś aktywny sexualnie?	YES-tesh ak-TYV-ni sek-soo-AL-n-ye?

Do you use condoms?	Czy używasz prezerwatsyu?	chi oo-ZHI-vash pre-ser-VATS-yoo?
Homosexual	Homoseksualista	ho-mo-sek-soo-a-LEES-ta

SYSTEMS REVIEW

Do you have...	Czy masz...?	chi mash...?

GENERAL

Fever	Gorączkę	gor-YACH-ke*ng*
Chills	Dreszcze	DRESH-che
Weight loss	Utratę wagi	oo-TRA-te*ng* VA-gee
Fatigue	Zmęczenie	z-me*ng*-CHEN-ee-yey
Sick contact	Kontakt z chorym	KON-takt z KHOR-im

HEENT

Sore throat	Ból gardła	bool GARD-wa
Runny nose	Katar	KA-tar
Nosebleed	Krew z nosa	krev z NO-sa
Ear pain	Ból ucha	bool OO-kha
Ear ringing	Dzwonienie ucha	j-vo-n-YE-n-ye OO-kha
Decreased hearing	Pogorszony słuch	po-gor-SHO-ni swookh

EYE

Eye pain	Ból oka	bool O-ka
Blurry vision	Niewyraźne widzenie	n-ye-vi-RAZH-ne vee-JE-nee-ye
Diplopia	Podwójne widzenie	pod-VOY-ne vee-JE-nee-ye

(cont.)

Foreign body sensation	Odczucie obcego ciała	ot-CHOO-chee-ye OB-tse-go tsee-YA-wa
Contact lenses	Szkła kontaktowe	shk-WA kon-tak-TO-ve
CARDIAC		
Chest pain	Ból klatki piersiowej	bool KLAT-ki p-yer-SHO-vey
Palpitations	Palpitacje (kołatanie)	pal-pi-TATS-ye (ko-wa-TAN-n-ye)
Orthopnea	Trudność w oddychaniu na leżąco	trood-NOSH-ch w od-di-KHAN-ee-yoo na le-ZHA*ng*-tso
Dyspnea on exertion	Ciężkie oddychanie z wysiłkiem	CHE*ng*-zh-KEE-ye od-di-KHA-nee-ye z vi-SHIW-kee-yem
Fainting (syncope)	Mdlenie	m-d-LEN-ee-ye
Leg swelling	Spuchniecie nóg	spookh-n-YE-che noog
How many pillows?	Ile poduszek?	EE-le po-DOO-shek?
PULMONARY		
Trouble breathing	Ciężko oddychać	CHE*ng*-zh-ko od-di-KHACH
SOB	Płytkie oddychanie	p-WIT-kee-ye od-di-KHA-nee-ye
Cough	Kaszel	KA-shel
Sputum	Flema	FLE-ma
Pain on inspiration	Ból podczas wdechu	bool POD-chas V-DE-khoo
Hemoptysis	Krwioplucie	K-R-vee-o-PLOO-che

GI		
Abdominal pain	Ból brzucha	bool B-ZHOO-kha
Nausea	Mdłość	m-d-LOSH-ch
Vomiting	Wymioty	vi-mee-O-ti
Vomiting blood	Wymioty z krwią	vi-mee-O-ti z K-R-vee-a*ng*
Coffee ground emesis	Wymioty w postaci zmielonej kawy	vi-mee-O-ti w pos-TA-chee z-m-ye-LO-ney KA-vi
Anorexia	Anorexia	a-no-REK-see-a
Diarrhea	Biegunka	b-ye-GOON-ka
Difficulty swallowing	Trudność w połykaniu	trood-NOSH-ch w po-wi-KA-nee-yoo
BRBPR	Jasno-czerwona krew w odbycie	YAS-no-cher-VO-na krev w od-BI-che
Melena	Czarna krew w odbycie	CHAR-na krev w od-BI-che
Pain after eating	Ból po jedzeniu	bool po ye-JE-nee-yoo
Worms	Robaki	ro-BA-kee
Constipation	Zatwardzenie	zat-vard-JEN-n-ye
GU		
Painful urination	Oddawanie moczu z bólem	od-da-VA-n-ye MO-choo z BOOL-em
Urgent urination	Nagłe oddawanie moczu	NAG-we od-da-VA-n-ye MO-choo
Frequent urination	Częste oddawanie moczu	CHE*ng*-ste od-da-WA-n-ye MO-choo
Bloody urination	Krew w moczu	krev v MO-choo

(cont.)

Discharge: vaginal/penile	Wydzielina z pochwy/penisa	vid-jee-el-EE-na z POKH-vi/pe-NEE-sa
PSYCH		
Anxiety	Lęk	le*ng*-k
Depression	Depresja	de-PRE-see-a
Suicidal thoughts	Myśli sambójcze	MISH-lee sam-BOOY-che
Homicidal thoughts	Myśli zabójcze	MISH-lee za-BOOY-che
Medication overdose	Przedawkowanie lekami	p-she-dav-ko-VA-n-ye le-KA-mee
Hear voices	Słyszenie głosów	swi-SHE-nee-ye gwo-SOOV
NEURO		
Headache	Ból głowy	bool GWO-vi
Worst headache of life	Najgorszy ból głowy	nay-GOR-shi BOOL GWO-vi
Weakness	Słabość	SWA-bosh-ch
Dizzy	Odurzony	o-door-ZHO-ni
What is your name?	Jak się nazywasz?	yak she*ng* na-zi-VASH?
Where are we?	Gdzie jesteśmy?	g-JE yes-TESH-mi
What is the year/month/date?	Jaki teraz jest rok / miesiąc / data?	YA-kee TER-az yest rok /m-YE-sha*ng*-ts / DA-ta
Bowel dysfunction	Dysfunkcja jelitowa	dis-FOONK-ts-ya ye-lee-TO-va
Bladder dysfunction	Dysfunkcja pęcherza	dis-FOONK-ts-ya p-ye-KHER-tsa
Photophobia	Światłowstręt	sh-v-YAT-lov-st-RE*ng*-T
Tingling/numbness	Zdrętwienie / martwota	z-dre*ng*t-v-YE-n-ye / mart-VO-ta

Polish—Polski

Decreased strength in... (See Body Part List)	Osłabienie...	os-wab-YE-nee-ye...
Seizure	Padaczka	pa-DACH-ka
Difficulty walking	Trudność w chodzeniu	TROOD-nosh-ch v kho-JEN-ee-yoo
Difficulty speaking	Trudność w mówieniu	TROOD-nosh-ch v moov-YE-nee-yoo
Spinning (vertigo)	Kręci sie w głowie	KREng-chee sh-ye v GLOV-ee- ye
Confusion	Dezorientacja	de-zor-ee-yen-TATS-ya
MISC		
Lump	Guz	gooz
Itching	Swędzenie	s-veng-JEN-ee-ye
Bruising	Sinienie	see-n-YE-n-ye
Rash	Wysypka	vi-SIP-ka
Swelling	Spuchnięcie	spookh-n-YEng-chee-ye
Jaundice (yellow skin)	Żółtaczka	zhoow-TACH-ka
GYNECOLOGIC		
Vaginal bleeding	Krwawienie z pochwy	k-r-vav-YE-nee-ye z POKH-vi
Heavy	Ciężki	CHEng-zh-kee
Irregular	Nieregularny	n-ye-re-goo-LAR-ni
Absent	Nieobecny	n-ye-o-BETS-ni
Vaginal discharge	Wydzielina z pochwy	vi-JE-lee-na z POKH-vi

(cont.)

Pelvic pain	Ból w miednicy	bool v m-yed-NEE-tsi
Rape	Gwałt	g-VALT
Pain with intercourse	Ból podczas stosunku	bool POD-chas sto-SOON-koo
Contraceptive	Antykoncepcyjny	AN-ti-kon-tsep-TSI-ni

OBSTETRIC

Are you pregnant?	Jesteś w ciąży?	YES-tesht v ch-YA*ng*-zhi?
LMP how many days ago?	Ile dni temu miałaś miesiączkę?	EE-le d-nee TE-moo mee-YA-wash m-ye-SHA*ng*CH-ke*ng*?
Times pregnant?	Ile razy byłaś w ciąży?	EE-le RA-zi BI-wash v ch-YA*ng*-zhi?
Times delivered?	Ile miałaś porodów?	EE-le mee-YA-wash po-ro-DOOV?
Miscarriage	Poronienie	po-ro-n-YE-n-ye
Abortion	Aborcja	a-BORTS-ya
Fluid leakage	Wyciekanie płynu	vi-chee-ye-KA-n-ye p-WE-noo
Contraction	Kontrakcja	kon-TRAKTS-ya
Fetal movement	Poruszanie płodu	po-roo-SHA-n-ye PWO-doo

TRAUMA

How many hours ago did you eat last?	Ile godzin temu miałeś ostatni posiłek? (to a man); Ile godzin temu miałaś ostatni posiłek? (to a woman)	EE-le GO-jeen TE-moo mee-YA-wesh os-TAT-nee po-SEE-wek? (to a man); EE-le GO-jeen TE-moo mee-YA-wash os-TAT-nee po-SEE-wek? (to a woman)

Lost consciousness?	Straciłeś przytomność? (to a man); Straciłaś przytomność? (to a woman)	stra-CHEE-wesh p-shi-TOM-nosh-ch? (to a man); stra-CHEE-wash p-shi-TOM-nosh-ch? (to a woman)
Tetanus within 5 years?	Szczepionka na tężec w ostatnich pięciu latach?	sh-che-pee-YON-ka na TYEng-zhets v o-STAT-neekh pee-YEng-chee-yoo LA-tach
PEDIATRIC		
How old?	Ile lat?	EE-le lat
Vaccines up to date?	Wszystkie szczepienia na czas?	v-SHIST-k-ye sh-chep-YE-nee-ya na chas
Urinating normally	Normalne oddawanie moczu?	nor-MAL-ne od-da-VA-nee-ye MO-choo
Taking liquids	Pije płyny / wody?	PEE-ye p-WY-ni / VO-dy
Increased crying	Częściejsze płacze?	cheng-sh-che-YE-she PWA-che?
Ingestion	Przyjmowanie pokarmu	p-shiy-mo-VA-n-ye po-KAR-moo
Foreign body	Obce ciało	OB-tse CHA-wo
Premature	Przedwczesne	p-SHED-v-CHES-n-ye
Birth complications	Komplikacje porodowe	kom-plee-KATS-ye po-ro-DO-ve
PHYSICAL EXAM/INSTRUCTION		
Sit down (please)	Usiądź (proszę)	oo-SHAng-j (PRO-sheng)
Lie down	Połóż się	po-WOOSH sh-yeng
Come here	Przyjdź tutaj	p-SHEEJ TOO-tay

(cont.)

Relax	Zrelaksuj się	z-re-LAK-sooy sh-ye*ng*
Don't move	Nie ruszaj się	n-ye ROO-shay sh-ye*ng*
Open your mouth	Otwórz usta	ot-VOORZ OO-sta
Say "ahh"	Powiedz "aaa"	PO-veej "aaa"
Swallow	Połknij	POW-k-neey
Breath deeply	Oddychaj głęboko	od-di-KHAY gle*ng*-BO-ko
Hold your breath	Nie oddychaj	n-ye o-di-KHAY
Cough	Kaszel	KA-shel
Push	Pchaj	p-KHAY
Pull	Ciągnij	chee-ya*ng*-NEE
Follow my fi*ng*er	Patrz na mój palec	PAT-zh na mooy PA-lets
Close your eyes	Zamknij oczy	ZAMK-neey O-chee
Smile	Uśmiechnij się	oosh-m-YESH-nee sh-ye
Can you feel this?	Czujesz to?	CHOO-yesh to?
Copy this (movement)	Powtórz to (ten ruch)	pov-TOORZ to (ten rookh)
I am going to put a finger in your rectum	Wsadzę palec w twój odbyt	v-SHA-je PA-lets v t-voy OD-bit
I am going to examine your vagina	Zbadam twoją pochwę	z-BA-dam t-VO-ya*ng* POKH-ve*ng*
REASSESSMENT		
Do you feel better?	Czujesz się lepiej?	CHOO-yesh she*ng* LE-pee-yey?

Polish—Polski

Do you feel worse?	Czujesz się gorzej?	CHOO-yesh sheng GOR-zey
PATIENT WORDS		
I hurt	Jestem w bólu / Boli	YES-tem v BOOL-oo / BO-lee
Help!	Pomóż!	po-MOOZ
Bathroom	Łazienka	wa-ZH-en-ka
Food	Żywność	zhiv-NOSH-ch
Water	Woda	VO-da
PROCEDURES & CONSENT		
You need...	Potrzebujesz / Musisz mieć	pot-ZHE-boo-yesh / MOO-seesh m-YECH
Injection	Zastrzyk	ZAST-zhik
Stiches	Szwy	sh-VI
Cast	Gips	geeps
Crutches	Kule	KOO-le
Perform surgery on the... (See Body Parts List)	Operacje na...	o-per-ATS-ye na...
The risks are...	Jest ryzyko...	YEST RI-zi-ko...
Bleeding	Krwawienia	kr-va-vee-YEN-ee-a
Infection	Infekcji	een-FEKTS-yee
Scar	Blizny	BLEEZ-ni
Repeat procedure	Powtórzenia zabiegu	pov-TOO-zhen-ee-ya za-b-YE-goo
Iodine	Jod	yod
Damage to your...(See Body Parts List)	Uszkodzenie...	oosh-ko-JE-nee-ye...
Sign here	Podpisz tutaj	POD-peesh TOO-tay

(cont.)

Polish—Polski

TESTS		
X-ray	Prześwietlenie	p-zhesh-svee-yet-LE-neeye
C.A.T. Scan	Tomografia komputerowa	to-mo-GRA-fee-ya kom-POO-ter-O-va
Ultrasound	Ultradźwięk (USG)	oo-TRAJ-vengk (oo-es-ge)
Catheterization/ bladder catheter	Cewnikowanie / pęcherzowy kateter	tsev-nee-ko-VA-n-ye / peng-kher-ZO-vi KA-ta-ter
Colonoscopy (from below)/ Endoscopy (from above)	Badanie okrężnicy	ba-DA-n-ye o-krengzh-NEE-tsi
Endoscopy	Endoskopia	en-do-SKO-pee-a
END OF LIFE		
Do you want us to…	Czy chcesz żebyśmy…	chi kh-tsesh zhe-BISH-mi…
Perform CPR	Resuscytacja Krążeniowo Oddechowa (RKO)	re-soos-tsi-TA-tsee-a krang-zhe-N-YO-ve od-de-KHO-va (er-ke-o)
Defibrillate	Defibrylować	de-feeb-ri-LO-vach
Intubate	Intubacja	een-too-BATS-ya
He/she is dead	On / Ona jest martwy/a	on (he) / ona (she) yest (is) MART-vy (masc) MART-va (fem)
We did all we could	Zrobiliśmy wszystko co w naszej mocy	z-ro-beel-EESH-mi v-SHIST-ko tso v na-shey MO-tsi
DISCHARGE		
You have…(See Medical Prob List)	Masz…	mash…

Polish—Polski

He/she is going to stay in the hospital	On / Ona zostanie w szpitalu	On (he) / Ona (she) zo-STA-n-ye v sh-pee-TAL-oo
Take "X" pills "Y" times a day for "Z" days	Bierz "X" tabletki "Y" razy dziennie przez "Z" dni	b-YESH "X" tab-LET-kee "Y" RA-zi dz-YEN-n-ye p-sed "Z" d-nee
Pills	Tabletki	tab-LET-kee
Antibiotics	Antybiotyki	AN-ti-bee-O-tee-kee
Before/after meals	Przed i po jedzeniu	p-zhed ee po ye-JEN-ee-yoo
Return to the ER if...	Powróć do szpitala jeżeli	pov-ROOCH do sh-pee-TA-la ye-ZHE-lee...
Follow up at "X" on "Y"	Powróć na badanie do "X" "Y"	pov-ROOCH na ba-DA-n-ye do "X" "Y"
You're welcome	Proszę	PRO-sheng
Goodbye	Dowidzenia	do-vee-JE-nee-a
MEDICAL PROBS		
AIDS/HIV	AIDS / HIV	AIDS / HIV (eyd-z / ha-ee-ve)
Anemia	Anemia	a-NE-mee-a
Arrhythmia	Arytmia	a-RIT-mee-a
Arthritis	Reumatyzm	re-oo-ma-TI-zim
Asthma	Astma	AST-ma
Bronchitis	Bronchit	bron-KHEET
Cancer	Rak	rak
Cirrhosis	Marskość	mar-SKOSH-ch
Cholesterol	Kolesterol	ko-les-te-ROL
Cold	Przeziębienie	p-zhezh-yeng-b-YE-n-ye

(cont.)

Constipation	Zatwardzenie	zat-var-JEN-n-ye
Cyst	Torbiel	TOR-bee-el
Diabetes	Cukrzyca	tsook-zhi-TSA
Dialysis	Dializa	dee-a-LEE-za
Diverticulitis	Infekcja jelit	een-FEK-TS-ya YEL-eet
Emphysema	Rozedma	ro-ZED-ma
Fibroids	Włókniak	v-WOOK-nee-ak
Fracture	Złamanie	zwa-MA-n-ye
Flu	Grypa	GRI-pa
Gallstones	Kamienie żółciowe	kam-YE-n-ye zhol-chi-O-ve
Gastritis/GERD	Nieżyt żąłądka	n-YE-zhit zha-WA*ng*D-ka
Hepatitis	Żółtaczka	zhool-TACH-ka
Heart attack	Atak serca	a-TAK SER-tsa
Heart disease	Choroba serca	kho-RO-ba SER-tsa
Heart failure	Niedomoga serca	n-ye-do-MO-ga SER-tsa
Hypertension	Nadciśnienie	na-chish-n-YE-n-ye
Indigestion	Niestrawność	n-ye-STRAV-nosh-ch
Kidney stone	Kamienie nerkowe	kam-YE-n-ye ner-KO-ve
Lupus	Toczeń	TO-chen
Migraine	Migrena	mee-GREN-a
Murmur	Szmer	sh-mer
Pacemaker	Stymulator serca	sti-moo-LA-tor SER-tsa
Pneumonia	Zapalenie płuc	za-pa-LE-n-ye p-woots

Polish—Polski 203

Seizures	Padaczka	pa-DACH-ka
STD	Choroby przekazywane drogą płciową	kho-RO-ba p-zhe-KA-zi-va-ne DRO-ga p-w-CHO-wang
Stroke	Wylew	VI-lev
Ulcer	Wrzód	v-ZHOOD
Ulcerative colitis	Wrzodowe zapalenie okrężnicy	v-zho-DO-ve z-pa-LEN-ee-ye o-krengzh-NEETS-i
UTI	Infekcja przewodów moczowych	een-FEKTS-ya p-zheh-VO-doov mo-CHO-vikh
BODY PARTS		
Abdomen	Brzuch	b-ZHOOKH
Ankle	Kostka	KOST-ka
Appendix	Wyrostek robaczkowy	vi-RO-stek ro-bach-KO-vi
Arm	Ramię	RAM-yeng
Artery	Arteria	ar-TER-ee-a
Back	Plecy	PLE-tsi
Bladder	Pęcherz	PEng-kherz
Blood	Krwawy	kr-VA-vi
Bone	Kość	KOSH-ch
Brain	Mózg	MOOZ-g
Breast	Pierś	p-YER-sh
Calf	Łydka	WID-ka
Chest	Klatka piersowa	KLAT-ka p-yer-SHO-va
Chin	Podbródek	pod-BROO-dek

(cont.)

Ear	Ucho	OO-kho
Elbow	Łokieć	WO-kee-ech
Eye	Oko	O-ko
Face	Twarz	t-VAR-z
Finger	Palec	PA-lets
Foot	Stopa	STO-pa
Hand	Ręka	RE*ng*-ka
Head	Głowa	GWO-va
Heart	Serce	SER-tse
Gallbladder	Żółciowy	zhoow-CHO-vi
Jaw	Szczęka	sh-CHE*ng*-ka
Joint	Staw	stav
Kidney	Nerka	NER-ka
Knee	Kolano	ko-LA-no
Leg	Noga	NO-ga
Liver	Wątroba	va*ng*-TRO-ba
Mouth	Usta	OO-sta
Muscle	Mięsień	mee-E*ng*-shen
Neck	Szyja	SHEE-ya
Nerve	Nerw	nerv
Nose	Nos	nos
Ovary	Jajnik	YAY-neek
Pancreas	Trzustka	t-ZHOOST-ka
Penis	Penis	PEN-ees
Prostate	Prostata	pro-STA-ta
Rectum	Odbytnica	od-bit-NEETS-a
Rib	Żebro	ZHE-bro

Polish—Polski

Shoulder	Bark	bark
Skin	Skóra	SKOO-ra
Spleen	Śledziona	sh-le-JEE-o-na
Spine	Kręgosłup	kreng-GO-swoop
Stomach	Żołądek	zho-WAng-dek
Teeth	Zęby	ZEng-bi
Testicle	Jądra	YAng-dra
Throat	Gardło	GARD-wo
Thyroid	Tarczyca	tar-CHI-tsa
Toe	Palec u nogi	PA-lets oo no-gee
Tonsils	Migdały	meeg-DA-wi
Tongue	Język	YEng-zik
Uterus	Macica	MA-chee-tsa
Vagina	Pochwa	POKH-va
Vein	Żyła	ZHI-wa
Wrist	Nadgarstek	nad-GAR-stek
NUMBERS		
How many (times)?	Ile (razy)?	EE-le RA-zi
0	Zero	ZE-ro
1	Jeden	YE-den
2	Dwa	d-VA
3	Trzy	t-ZHI
4	Cztery	ch-TE-ri
5	Pięć	p-YEng-ch
6	Sześć	SHESH-ch
7	Siedem	SHE-dem

(cont.)

8	Osiem	O-shem
9	Dziewięć	JE-vee-yengch
10	Dziesięć	JE-shee-Engch
11	Jedenaście	ye-den-ASH-ch-ye
20	Dwadzieścia	d-va-je-YESH-ch-ya
30	Trzydzieści	t-zhi-je-YESH-chi
40	Czterdzieści	ch-ter-je-YESH-chi
50	Pięćdziesiąt	p-YEng-ch-ji-sh-angt
60	Sześćdziesiąt	sh-esh-ch-JE-sh-angt
70	Siedemdziesiąt	sh-e-dem-JE-sh-angt
80	Osiemdziesiąt	o-shem-JE-sh-angt
90	Dziewięćdziesiąt	Jeng-vee-yengch-je-SH-YAngt
100	Sto	sto

Portuguese—Português

WORD/PHRASE	TRANSLATION	ENGLISH PRONUNCIATION
Portuguese	Português	por-too-GEYSH
INTRODUCTION & REGISTRATION		
Hello	Oi	OY
I am a doctor / nurse	Sou médico / enfermeiro	SO-oo ME-jee-ko / en-fer-MEY-ro
What is your name?	Qual é seu nome?	KWA-le SE-oo NO-mee
Who is your doctor?	Quem é seu médico?	kem e SEE-oo ME-jee-ko?
How old are you?	Quantos anos têm você?	KWAN-tos A-nos tem vo-SE?
Birthdate?	Data de nascimento?	DA-ta jee na-see-MEN-too
Telephone number?	O número de telefone?	o NOO-me-ro jee te-le-FO-ne
Address?	Endereço	EN-de-re-so
Social security number?	Número de Seguro Social	NOO-me-ro jee se-GOO-ro so-see-YA-oo
Insurance?	Seguro	se-GOO-ro
BASICS		
Do you understand?	Você compreende?	vo-SE com-PREN-jee?
Yes	Sim	seem
No	Não	NA-oo
Please	Por Favor	por FA-vo
Thank you	Obrigado	o-bree-GA-doo
Sorry	Desculpa	des-KOOL-pa
I don't understand	Eu não compreendo	E-oo NA-oo com-PREN-doo

(cont.)

English	Portuguese	Pronunciation
Repeat	Fale novamente	FA-le no-va-MEN-chee
Speak slowly	Fale lentamente	FA-le len-ta-MEN-chee
Answer "yes" or "no"	Responda "sim" ou "não"	khes-PON-da "SEEM" o "NA-oo"
Here	Aqui	a-KEE
This	Isto	EES-too
It's alright (consoling)	Tudo está bem	TOO-doo es-TA bem
I'll be right back	Não tardo em voltar	NA-oo TAR-do em vol-TAR

GENERAL

English	Portuguese	Pronunciation
What's wrong?	Qual é o problema?	KWA-oo E oo pro-BLE-ma?
Pain	Dor	dor
Do you have pain?	Você tem dor?	vo-SE tem dor?
Does the pain radiate?	A dor vai a outro lugar?	a dor VAY a O-oo-troo loo-GAR?
Where (show me)	Onde	ON-jee
Gone now	é ido	e EE-doo
Still present	Ainda presente	a-EEN-da pre-SEN-chee
Sudden/gradual onset	Ataque súbito /gradual	a-TA-ke SOO-bee-too / gra-doo-A-oo
What bothers you the most?	O que o incomoda mais	oo ke o een-co-MO-da MA-ees
Why did you come today?	Por que você vêm hoje	por-KE vo-SE vem O-zhe

QUALITY

English	Portuguese	Pronunciation
If '0' is no pain and 10 is maximum pain, what number do you have now?	Se 0 não for nenhuma dor, e 10 é a dor máxima, que número você tem agora?	se ZE-ro NA-oo for nen-YOO-ma dor, e dez e a dor MA-zee-ma, ke NOO-me-ro vo-SE tem a-GO-ra?
Burning	Ardência	ar-DEN-see-a

Constant	Constante	kon-STAN-chee
Dull	Vagaroso (não agudo)	va-ga-RO-so (NA-oo a-GOO-doo)
Intermittent	Intermitente	een-TER-mee-ten-chee
Pressure	Pressão	pre-SA-oo
Severe	Severo	se-VE-roo
Sharp/prickly pains	Agudo / espinhoso	a-GOO-doo / es-peen-YO-soo
Throbbing	Batimento	ba-chee-MEN-too
ASSOCIATED SYMPTOMS		
Onset during... (before/after)	Ataque durante... (antes / depois)	a-ta-ke doo-RAN-chee... (AN-tes / dee-PO-EESH)
Worse (with...)	Pior com...	PEE-or com...
Better (with...)	Melhor com...	me-lee-OR com...
Cough	Tosse	TO-see
Deep breath	Respiração profunda	khes-pee-ra-SA-oo pro-FOON-da
Emotional upset	Pertubaçao emocional	PER-too-ba-SA-oo e-mo-see-o-NA-oo
Food	Comida	ko-MEE-da
Movement	Movimento	mo-vee-MEN-too
Nothing	Nada	NA-da
Positioning	Posicionamento	po-see-so-na-MEN-too
Rest	Descanso	des-KAN-soo
Walking	Andar	an-DAR
TIME COURSE		
For how long?	Quanto tempo faz?	KWAN-to TEM-po faz?
Today	Hoje	O-zhe

(cont.)

Yesterday	Ontem	ON-tem
How many...	Quantos	KWAN-tos
Months/weeks/days/hours/seconds	Meses / semanas / dias / horas / segundos	ME-zes / se-MA-nas / JEE-as / O-ras / se-GOON-dos
Still present?	Ainda presente?	a-EEN-da pre-SEN-chee
Gone now?	é ido?	e EE-doo
How long did it last? (See Number List)	Quanto tempo ele durou?	KWAN-to TEM-po E-lee doo-RO-OO?
Have you had this before?	Você teve isto antes?	vo-SE TE-ve EES-to AN-chees
How many times?	Quantas vezes?	KWAN-tas VE-zes?
When was the last time?	Quando foi a última vez	KWAN-doo foy a OOL-chee-ma veyz
New	Novo	NO-voo
Old	Velho	VEL-yo
CONTEXT		
Did you...?	Você..?	vo-SE
fall	caiu	ka-ee-OO
trip	tropeçou	tro-peh-SO-oo
faint	desmaiou	des-ma-YO-oo
twist	torseu	tor-SE-oo
get hit	foi ferido	FOY fe-REE-do
get burned	se queimou	se key-MO-oo
get assaulted	foi agredido	FOY a-gre-JEE-do
get bitten (human/dog/cat/insect)	foi mordido	FOY mor-DEE-do
PAST MEDICAL HISTORY		
Take medication?	Toma a medicação?	TO-ma a me-jee-ca-SA-oo

(aspirin/antibiotics)	Aspirina, antibióticos	as-pee-REE-na, an-chee-bee-O-chee-koos
Do you have (See also Medical Problem List)…	Você tem	vo-SE tem
allergies	Alergias	a-LER-jee-as
medical problems	Problemas médicos	prob-LE-mas ME-jee-koos
Do you have problems of the… (see Body Parts List)	…problemas de	…prob-LE-mas jee
SURGICAL HISTORY		
Have you had surgery?	Você teve cirurgia	vo-SE te-ve see-roo-JEE-a
Surgery on/"to remove"…(see Body Parts List)	Cirugia em..	see-roo-JEEA em…
SOCIAL HISTORY		
Smoke?	Fuma?	FOO-ma?
Drink?	Bebe?	BE-be?
Take drugs?	Droga-se?	DRO-ga se?
Recent travel?	Viagem recente?	vi-A-jem he-SEN-chee?
Are you sexually active?	Você é sexualmente ativo?	vo-SE e se-shoo-al-MEN-chee a-CHEE-voo?
Do you use condoms?	Você usa preservativos?	vo-SE OO-zha pre-ser-va-CHEE-voos?
Homosexual	Homossexual	o-mo-sek-soo-A-oo
SYSTEMS REVIEW		
Do you have…	Você tem…	vo-SE tem…
GENERAL		
Fever	Febre	FE-bre

(cont.)

Chills	Calafrios	KA-la-FREE-oos
Weight loss	Perda de Peso	PER-da jee PE-zo
Fatigue	Fatiga	FA-tee-ga
Sick contact	Contato doente	kon-TA-too do-EN-chee
HEENT		
Sore throat	Garganta dolorida	gar-GAN-ta do-lo-REE-da
Runny nose	Nariz escorre	na-REEZ es-KO-re
Nosebleed	O nariz sangra	o na-REEZ SAN-gra
Ear pain	Dor de ouvido	dor jee O-oo-VEE-doo
Ear ringing	Zumbido no ouvido	ZOOM-bee-doo noo o-oo-VEE-doo
Decreased hearing	Redução de audição	khe-doo-SA-oo jee a-oo-jee-SA-o
EYE		
Eye pain	Dor de olho	dor jee O-lee-o
Blurry vision	Visão embaçada	vee-SA-o EM-ba-sa-da
Diplopia	Diplopia	jee-plo-PEE-a
Foreign body sensation	Sensação de corpo estranito	sen-sa-SA-oo jee KOR-poo es-TRAN-nee-too
Contact lenses	Lentes de contato	LEN-cheez jee kon-TA-to
CARDIAC		
Chest pain	Dor no peito	DOR noo PE-ee-to
Palpitations	Palpitações	pal-PEE-ta-so-eens
Orthopnea	Orthopnea	or-top-NEE-a
Dyspnea on exertion	Brevidade de respiração em esforço	bre-vee-DA-jee jee khes-PEE-ra-SA-oo em es-FOR-so
Fainting (syncope)	Desmaiar	des-MAY-ar

Leg swelling	Inchação de perna	een-sha-SA-oo jee PER-na
How many pillows?	Quantos travesseiros?	KWAN-tos tra-ve-SAY-ros

PULMONARY

Trouble breathing	Problema com respiração	pro-BLE-ma kom hes-PEE-ra-SA-oo
SOB	Brevidade de respiração	bre-vee-DA-jee jee hes-PEE-ra-SA-oo em es-FOR-so
Cough	Tosse	TO-see
Sputum	Substância segredas	soob-STAN-see-a se-GRE-das
Pain on inspiration	Dor em inspiração	dor em een-SPEE-ra-SA-o
Hemoptysis	Tossir sangue	to-SEER SAN-gee

GI

Abdominal pain	Dor abdominal	dor ab-do-mee-NA-oo
Nausea	Náusea	NA-oo-see-a
Vomiting	Vômito	VO-mee-to
Vomiting blood	Vômito com sangue	VO-mee-to com SAN-gee
Coffee ground emesis	Vômito de cor vermelho escuro	VO-mee-to jee kor ver-ME-lee-o es-KOO-roo
Anorexia	Anorexia	a-no-REK-see-A
Diarrhea	Diarréia	jee-a-KHE-a
Difficulty swallowing	Dificuldade engolir	jee-FEE-kool-DA-jee en-GO-leer
BRBPR	Sangue vivo por reto	SAN-gee VEE-vo por KHE-too
Melena	Excremento preto por causa de sangue	eks-kre-MEN-to PRE-to por KA-oo-sa jee SAN-gee

(cont.)

Pain after eating	Dor depois de comer	DOR de-PO-ees jee CO-mer
Worms	Vermes	VER-mees
Constipation	Constipação	KONS-chee-pa-SA-oo

GU

Painful urination	Urinação dolorosa	OO-ree-na-SA-oo do-lo-RO-sa
Urgent urination	Urinação urgente	OO-ree-na-SA-oo oor-ZHEN-chee
Frequent urination	Urinação freqüente	OO-ree-na-SA-oo fre-koo-EN-chee
Bloody urination	Urinação sangrenta	OO-ree-na-SA-oo san-GREN-ta
Discharge: vaginal/penile	Descarga:vaginal/ de pênis	des-KAR-ga: VA-zhee-NAU/ jee PE-nees

PSYCH

Anxiety	Ansiedade	AN-see-e-DA-dee
Depression	Depressão	de-pre-SA-o
Suicidal thoughts	Pensamentos suicidas	PEN-sa-MEN-tos soo-ee-SEE-das
Homicidal thoughts	Pensamentos homicidas	PEN-sa-MEN-tos o-mee-SEE-das
Medication overdose	Dose excessiva de medicação	DO-se ex-se-SEE-va jee ME-dee-ka-SA-oo
Hear voices	Ouve vozes?	OU-vee VO-zees

NEURO

Headache	Dor de cabeça	DOR jee ka-BE-za
Worst headache of life	A pior dor de cabeça de vida	a PEE-or dor jee ka-BE-za jee VEE-da
Weakness	Fraqueza	fra-KE-za
Dizzy	Tontura	ton-TOO-ra

What is your name?	Como se chama você?	KO-mo se SHA-ma vo-SE?
Where are we?	Onde nós estamos?	ON-jee nos es-TA-mos?
What is the year/month/date?	Qual é o ano, o mês, data?	KWA-oo E oo A-no, oo MES, a DA-ta?
Bowel dysfunction	Disfunção de intestino	jees-foon-SA-oo jee in-tes-CHEE-no
Bladder dysfunction	Disfunção de bexiga	jees-foon-SA-oo jee be-SHEE-ga
Photophobia	Fotofobia	fo-to-FO-bee-a
Tingling/numbness	Formigar/entorpecida	FOR-mee-gar / en-tor-pe-SEE-da
Decreased strength in…(See Body Parts List)	Força reduzida em…	FOR-sa he-doo-SEE-da em…
Seizure	Convulsões	kon-vool-SO-ens
Difficulty walking	Tem dificuldade para andar?	TEM dee-FEE-kool-TA-jee pa-ra an-DAR?
Difficulty speaking	Tem dificuldade para falar?	TEM dee-FEE-kool-TA-jee pa-ra fa-LAR?
Spinning (vertigo)	Vertigens	VER-tee-zhens
Confusion	Confusão	kon-foo-SA-oo
MISC		
Lump	Massa	MA-sa
Itching	Coceira	ko-SE-ee-ra
Bruising	Hematoma	E-ma-TO-ma
Rash	Borbulha	bor-BOO-lee-a
Swelling	Inchação	een-sha-SA-oo
Jaundice (yellow skin)	Icterícia	eek-te-REE-see-a

(cont.)

GYNECOLOGIC		
Vaginal bleeding	Hemorragia vaginal	E-mo-kha-GEE-a VA-zhee-NA-oo
Heavy	Pesada	pe-ZA-da
Irregular	Irregular	ee-KHE-goo-LA
Absent	Ausente	a-oo-SEN-chee
Vaginal discharge	Descarga vaginal	des-KAR-ga VA-zhee-NAU
Pelvic pain	Dor pélvica	DOR PEL-vee-ka
Rape	Assaltado sexualmente	a-sal-TA-doo SEX-soo-al-MEN-chee
Pain with intercourse	Dor com sexo	DOR kom SEK-so
Contraceptive	Contraceptivo	KON-tra-sep-CHEE-vo
OBSTETRIC		
Are you pregnant?	Você está grávida?	vo-SE es-TA GRA-vee-da?
LMP how many days ago?	Data de última menstruação?	DA-ta jee OOL-chee-ma mens-troo-a-SA-oo?
Times pregnant?	Quantas vezes grávies?	KWAN-tas VE-zes GRA-ve-ees?
Times delivered?	Quantas vezes dau a luz?	KWAN-tas VE-zes DA-oo a LOOZ?
Miscarriage	Perder o bebê	PER-der o be-BE
Abortion	Aborto	a-BOR-to
Fluid leakage	Escoa o fluido	es-KO-a o FLOO-ee-do
Contraction	Contração	kon-tra-SA-o
Fetal movement	Movimento fetal	MO-vee-MEN-too fe-TA-oo
TRAUMA		
How many hours ago did you eat last?	Que horas você comeu?	ke O-ras vo-SE ko-ME-oo?

Lost consciousness?	Você perdeu a consciência?	vo-SE per-DE-oo a con-SEN-see-a
Tetanus within 5 years?	Tétano dentro de 5 anos passados?	TE-ta-noo DEN-troo jee SEEN-koo A-nos pa-SA-dos?
PEDIATRIC		
How old?	Quantos anos?	KWAN-tos A-nos
Vaccines up to date?	As suas vacinas até data?	as SOO-as va-SEE-nas A-te DA-ta
Urinating normally	Urinar normalmente?	oo-ree-NAR nor-mal-MEN-chee
Taking liquids	Toma líquidos	TO-ma LEE-kee-dos
Increased crying	Chorando mais que o normal?	sho-RAN-doo MA-ees ke o nor-MA-OO?
Ingestion	Ingestão	een-zhes-TA-oo
Foreign body	Corpo estranho	KOR-po es-TRA-nho
Premature	Prematuro	pre-ma-TOO-ro
Birth complications	Complicações de nascimento	kom-PLEE-ka-SO-ens jee NA-see-MEN-too
PHYSICAL EXAM/INSTRUCTION		
Sit down (please)	Sente-se	SEN-te-se
Lie down	Deitar	de-ee-TAR
Come here	Venha aqui	VEN-ya a-KEE
Relax	Relaxe	khe-LAK-se
Don't move	Não mover	NA-oo mo-VER
Open your mouth	Abra a sua boca	A-bra a SOO-a BO-ka
Say "ahh"	Diga "ahh"	JEE-ga "ahh"
Swallow	Engula	en-GOO-la

(cont.)

Breath deeply	Respira profundamente	khes-PEE-ra pro-FOON-da-MEN-chee
Hold your breath	Mantenha a sua respiração	man-TE-nha a SOO-a khes-PEE-ra-SA-oo
Cough	Tosse	TO-see
Push	Empurre	em-POO-he
Pull	Puxe	POO-she
Follow my finger	Siga o meu dedo	SEE-ga o ME-oo DE-doo
Close your eyes	Feche os seus olhos	FE-she os SE-oos O-lee-os
Smile	Sorria	so-KHEE-a
Can you feel this?	Você pode sentir isto?	vo-SE PO-dee sen-TEER EES-too?
Copy this (movement)	Copie este movimento	KO-pee-e ES-chee mo-vee-MEN-too
I am going to put a finger in your rectum	Colocarei um dedo no seu reto	ko-LO-ka-RE-ee oom DE-doo noo SE-oo HE-too
I am going to examine your vagina	Examinarei a sua vagina	EX-sa-mee-na-RE-ee a soo-a va-ZHEE-na

REASSESSMENT

Do you feel better?	Você sente-se melhor?	vo-SE SEN-te-se me-lee-OR?
Do you feel worse?	Você sente-se pior?	vo-SE SEN-te-se pee-OR?

PATIENT WORDS

I hurt	Tenho dor	TE-nyo DOR
Help!	Socorro!	so-KO-kho!
Bathroom	Banheiro	ba-N-YE-ee-roo
Food	Comida	ko-MEE-da
Water	Água	A-goo-a

PROCEDURES & CONSENT		
You need...	Você precisa...	vo-SE pre-CEE-sa...
Injection	Uma injeção	OO-ma EEN-zhe-SA-oo
Stiches	Pontos de costura	PON-toos jee kos-TOO-ra
Cast	Gêsso	JE-so
Crutches	Muletas	moo-LE-tas
Perform surgery on the... (See Body Parts List)	Precisará de cirurgia em...	pre-SEE-sa-RA jee see-roo-JEE-a em...
The risks are...	Os riscos incluem	os KHEES-koos een-KLOO-em
Bleeding	Hemorragia	e-mo-kha-GEE-a
Infection	Infecção	een-fek-SA-oo
Scar	Cicatriz	SEE-ka-treez
Repeat procedure	Repetir o procedimento	KHE-pe-teer o pro-se-jee-MEN-to
Iodine	Iodo	ee-o-do
Damage to your... (See Body Part List)	Dano ao...	DA-noo a-oo...
Sign here	Assine aqui	a-SEE-ne a-KEE
TESTS		
X-ray	Radiografias	KHA-jee-o-gra-FEE-as
C.A.T. Scan	Tomografia computado	TO-mo-gra-FEE-a kom-poo-TA-doo
Ultrasound	Ultra-som	OOL-tra-som
Catheterization/ bladder catheter	Cateter de bexiga	KA-te-ter jee be-SHEE-ga
Colonoscopy (from below)/Endoscopy (from above)	Colonoscopia	KO-lo-nos-ko-PEE-a

(cont.)

| Endoscopy | Endoscopia | EN-dos-ko-PEE-a |

END OF LIFE

Do you want us to…	Você quer que nós…	vo-SE KER ke nos…
Perform CPR	Executemos ressuscitação cardiopulmonar	EK-ze-koo-TE-mos khe-soo-SEE-ta-SA-oo KAR-dee-o-POOL-mo-nar
Defibrillate	Chocar	sho-KAR
Intubate	Intubar	een-too-BAR
He/she is dead	Ele está morto, ela está morta	E-lee es-TA MOR-too, E-la es-TA MOR-ta
We did all we could	Fizemos todo que poderíamos	fee-ZE-mos TO-doo ke po-de-REE-a-mos

DISCHARGE

You have…(See Medical Prob List)	Você tem…	vo-SE tem
He/she is going to stay in the hospital	Ele/Ela deve permanecer no hospital	E-lee/E-la DE-vee per-MA-ne-ser noo hos-pee-TAU
Take "X" pills "Y" times a day for "Z" days	Tome "X" pílula "Y" vezes por dia durante "Z" dias	TO-mee "X" PEE-loo-la "Y" VE-zees po JEE-a doo-RAN-chee "Z" JEE-as
Pills	Pílula	PEE-loo-la
Antibiotics	Antibióticos	an-CHEE-bee-O-chee-koos
Before/after meals	Antes/depois de comer	AN-tes/ dee-PO-ees jee ko-ME
Return to the ER if…	Volte à Sala de Emergência se…	VOL-te SA-la jee e-mer-zhen-SEE-a se…
Follow up at "X" on "Y"	Volte para "X" em "Y"	VOL-te PA-ra "X" em "Y"
You're welcome	De nada	jee NA-da

Goodbye	Adeus	A-de-oos
MEDICAL PROBS		
AIDS/HIV	Síndrome de Imunode-ficiência Humana	SEEN-dro-mee jee ee-mee-oo-no-dee-fee-SEN-see-a oo-MA-na
Anemia	Anemia	a-ne-MEE-A
Arrhythmia	Pulso irregular	POOL-soo EE-khe-goo-la
Arthritis	Artrite	AR-tree-chee
Asthma	Asma	AS-ma
Bronchitis	Bronquite	BRON-kee-chee
Cancer	Cancer	KAN-ser
Cirrhosis	Cirrose	see-KHO-see
Cholesterol	Colesterol	ko-LES-te-khol
Cold	Influenza	een-floo-EN-za
Constipation	Constipação	kons-tee-pa-SA-oo
Cyst	Cisto	SEES-too
Diabetes	Diabete	JEE-a-BE-chee
Dialysis	Diálise	jee-A-lee-see
Diverticulitis	Diverticulitis	jee-ver-chee-koo-LEE-chees
Emphysema	Enfisema	en-fee-ZE-ma
Fibroids	Fibroma	fee-BRO-ma
Fracture	Fratura	fra-TOO-ra
Flu	Influenza	een-floo-EN-za
Gallstones	Cálculos biliares	KAL-koo-loos BEE-lee-A-res
Gastritis/GERD	Gastrite	gas-TREE-chee

(cont.)

Hepatitis	Hepatite	he-pa-TEE-chee
Heart attack	Ataque de coração	a-TA-ke jee ko-ra-SA-oo
Heart disease	Doença de coração	do-EN-sa jee ko-ra-SA-oo
Heart failure	Falência do coração	fa-LEN-cee-a doo ko-ra-SA-oo
Hypertension	Hipertensão	EE-per-ten-SA-oo
Indigestion	Indigestão	EEN-dee-zhes-TA-oo
Kidney stone	Pedra de rim	PE-dra jee kheem
Lupus	Lupus	LOO-poos
Migraine	Dor de cabeça [migraine]	DOR jee ka-BE-za [migraine]
Murmur	Murmúrio	moo-MOO-ree-oo
Pacemaker	Marca passo	MAR-ka PA-zhoo
Pneumonia	Pneumonia	NE-oo-mo-NEE-a
Seizures	Convulsões	kon-vool-SO-ens
STD	Doença sexualmente transmitida	do-EN-sa jee sek-SOO-aoo-MEN-chee TRANS-mee-CHEE-da
Stroke	Ataque cerebral	a-TA-ke se-re-BRA-oo
Ulcer	Úlcera	OOL-se-ra
Ulcerative colitis	Colite ulcerativa	ko-LEE-chee OOL-se-ra-CHEE-va
UTI	Infecção urinária	EEN-fek-SA-oo oo-ree-NA-ree-a
BODY PARTS		
Abdomen	Abdome	ab-DO-mee
Ankle	Tornozelo	tor-no-ZE-lo
Appendix	Apêndice	a-PEN-dee-se
Arm	Braço	BRA-so

Artery	Artéria	ar-TE-ree-a
Back	Costas	KOS-tas
Bladder	Bexiga	be-SHEE-ga
Blood	Sangue	SAN-gee
Bone	Osso	O-so
Brain	Cérebro	SE-re-broo
Breast	Seios	se-EE-os
Calf	Barriga da perna	ba-REE-ga da PER-na
Chest	Peito	PE-ee-too
Chin	Queixo	KE-ee-zhoo
Ear	Orelha	o-RE-lee-a
Elbow	Cotovelo	ko-to-VE-loo
Eye	Olho	O-lee-o
Face	Cara	KA-ra
Finger	Dedo	DE-doo
Foot	Pé	pe
Hand	Mão	ma-oo
Head	Cabeça	ka-BE-za
Heart	Coração	ko-ra-SA-oo
Gallbladder	Vesícula biliar	ve-SEE-koo-la bee-lee-ar
Jaw	Maxila	MAK-see-la
Joint	Articulaçao	ar-TEE-koo-la-SA-oo
Kidney	Rim	kheem
Knee	Joelho	zho-E-lee-o
Leg	Perna	PER-na

(cont.)

Liver	Fígado	FEE-ga-do
Mouth	Boca	BO-ka
Muscle	Músculo	MOOS-koo-lo
Neck	Pescoço	pes-KO-zo
Nerve	Nervo	NER-vo
Nose	Nariz	na-REEZ
Ovary	Ovário	o-VA-ree-o
Pancreas	Pâncreas	PAN-kre-as
Penis	Pênis	PE-nees
Prostate	Próstata	PROS-ta-ta
Rectum	Reto	HE-too
Rib	Costela	kos-TE-la
Shoulder	Ombro	OM-bro
Skin	Pele	PE-le
Spleen	Baço	BA-so
Spine	Espinha	es-PEE-nha
Stomach	Estômago	es-TO-ma-go
Teeth	Dentes	DEN-chees
Testicle	Testículo	tes-TEE-koo-lo
Throat	Garganta	gar-GAN-ta
Thyroid	Tireóide	chee-ree-O-dee
Toe	Dedo do Pé	DE-doo doo PE
Tonsils	Amígdalas	a-MEEG-da-las
Tongue	Língua	LEEN-goo-a
Uterus	Útero	OO-te-ro
Vagina	Vagina	VA-zhee-na
Vein	Veia	VE-ee-a

Wrist	Pulso	POOL-so
NUMBERS		
How many (times)?	Quantas vezes?	KWAN-tas VE-zees?
0	Zero	ZE-roo
1	Um	oom
2	Dois	do-ees
3	Três	trez
4	Quatro	koo-A-tro
5	Cinco	SEEN-koo
6	Seis	SE-ees
7	Sete	SE-chee
8	Oito	O-ee-to
9	Nove	NO-vee
10	Dez	des
11	Onze	ON-zee
20	Vinte	VEEN-chee
30	Trinta	TREEN-ta
40	Quarenta	koo-a-REN-ta
50	Cinqüenta	seen-koo-EN-ta
60	Sessenta	se-ZHEN-ta
70	Setenta	se-TEN-ta
80	Oitenta	oee-TEN-ta
90	Noventa	no-VEN-ta
100	Cem	sem

Russian—Русский язык

WORD/PHRASE	TRANSLATION	ENGLISH PRONUNCIATION
Russian	Русский язык	ROOS-kee ya-ZIK
INTRODUCTION & REGISTRATION		
Hello	здравствуйте	z-DRAST-vooy-t-ye
I am a doctor / nurse	Я врач / медсестра (fem), медбрат (masc)	ya v-RACH / m-yed-sees-TRA (fem) / m-yed-BRAT (masc)
What is your name?	Как вас зовут?	kak vas zu-VOOT?
Who is your doctor?	Кто ваш врач?	k-TO vash v-RACH?
How old are you?	Сколько вам лет?	SKOL-ku vam L-YET?
Birthday?	Дата рождения	DA-ta ruzh-D-YE-nee-ya
Telephone number?	Номер телефона?	NO-meer tee-lee-FO-na
Address?	Адрес?	a-DR-YES
Social security number?	Ноумер социального обеспечения	NO-meer su-tsee-YAL-nu-vu u-b-yees-P-YE-ch-yen-nee-yu
Insurance?	Страхование	stra-khu-VAN-ee-ye
BASICS		
Do you understand?	Вы понимаете?	vi pu-nee-MA-ye-t-ye?
Yes	Да	DA
No	Нет	N-YET
Please	Пожалуйста	pu-ZHA-looy-sta
Thank you	Спасибо	spa-SEE-bu

(cont.)

Sorry	Извините	eez-vee-NEE-t-ye
I don't understand	Я не понимаю	ya nee pu-nee-MA-yoo
Repeat	Повторите	puv-tu-REE-t-ye
Speak slowly	Говорите медленно	gu-vu-REE-t-ye M-YED-leen-nu
Answer "yes" or "no"	Ответте «да» или «нет»	ut-VEE-t-ye "DA" EE-lee "N-YET"
Here	Здесь	z-D-YES
This	Это	E-tu
It's alright (consoling)	Всё в порядке	f-S-YO v pa-RYAD-kee
I'll be right back	Я сейчас вернусь	ya see-CHAS veer-NOOS

GENERAL

What's wrong?	Что с вами?	sh-TO s VA-mee
Pain	Боль	bol
Do you have pain?	У вас что-то болит?	oo vas sh-TO-tu bu-LEET?
Does the pain radiate?	боль куда-то отдаёт?	bol koo-DA-tu ut-da-YOT?
Where (show me)	Где/ куда? Покажите мене.	g-D-YE (where)/koo-DA (to where)? pu-ku-ZHEE-t-ye meen-YE
Gone now	Сейчас нет.	see-CHAS N-YET
Still present	Ещё есть	yeesh-CH-YO YES-t
Sudden/gradual onset	началось внезапно/ постепенно	na-cha-LOS v-nee-ZAP-nu / pu-stee-PYEN-nu
What bothers you the most?	Что вам мешает больше всего?	sh-TO vam mee-SHA-yet BOL-sh-ye f-sye-VO?

Why did you come today?	Почему пришли Вы сегодня?	pu-chee-MOO preesh-LEE see-VOD-n-ya?
QUALITY		
If '0' is no pain and 10 is maximum pain, what number do you have now?	Если «ноль» значит не болит, и «десять» значит максимальная боль, которой номер у вас сейчас?	YES-lee "nol" z-NA-cheet nee bu-LEET, ee "D-YES-s-yat" z-NA-cheet mak-see-MAL-na-ya bol, ku-TO-ree NOO-m-yer YES-t oo vas see-CHAS?
Burning	Жжёт?	ZHOT?
Constant	Постоянная?	pu-stu-YAN-na-ya
Dull	Тупая?	too-PA-ya
Intermittent	с перерывами?	s pee-R-YE-ri-va-mee
Pressure	Давит?	du-VEET?
Severe	Сильная?	SEEL-na-ya
Sharp/prickly pains	Острая?	OS-tra-ya
Throbbing	Колющая?	ku-L-YOOSH-cha-ya
ASSOCIATED SYMPTOMS		
Onset during... (before/after)	Начиналось во время...(перед/после)	na-chee-NA-lus vu v-R-YEM-ya (P-YE-reed/ POS-lee)
Worse (with...)	Хуже когда...	KHOO-zh-ye kug-DA...
Better (with...)	Лучше когда...	LOOCH-sh-ye kug-DA...
Cough	Кашель/кашляете	KA-shel / KASH-l-ya-ye-t-ye
Deep breath	Вдыхаете глубоко	v-di-KHA-ye-t-ye gloo-bu-KO

(cont.)

Emotional upset	Вы расстроенные?	vi ras-STRO-ye-nee-ye
Food	Во время еды / когда вы едите	vu v-R-YEM-ya ye-DI / kug-DA vi ye-DEE-t-ye
Movement	Перемещение / боль перемещается	Pee-ree-me-SH-YE-nee-ye / BOL pee-ree-mee-SHA-yet-su
Nothing	Ничего / ничего не делаете	nee-chee-VO / nee-chee-VO nee D-YE-la-ye-t-ye
Positioning	Меняете положение	meen-YA-ye-t-ye pu-lu-ZH-YEN-nee-ye
Rest	Во время отдыха / Когда отдыхаете	Vu v-R-YEM-ya OT-di-kha / kug-DA ut-di-KHA-ye-t-ye
Walking	Ходите	KHO-dee-t-ye
TIME COURSE		
For how long?	Как долго?	kak DOL-gu?
Today	Сегодня	see-VOD-n-ya
Yesterday	Вчера	f-ch-ye-RA
How many...	Сколько...	SKOL-ku...
Months/weeks/days/hours/seconds	месяцев / недель / дней / часов / секунд	M-YES-yu-ts-yef (months) / nee-D-YEL (weeks) / d-N-YEY (days) / chu-ZOF (hours) / see-KOONT (seconds)
Still present?	Ещё болит?	yee-SHO bu-LEET?
Gone now?	Сейчас не болит?	see-CHAS nee bu-LEET?
How long did it last? (See Numbers List)	Сколько времени продолжалось?	SKOL-ku v-R-YE-m-ye-nee pru-dul-ZHA-lus?

Russian—Русский язык

Have you had this before?	У вас это раньше случалось?	oo vas E-tu RAN-she sloo-CHA-lus?
How many times?	Сколько раз?	SKOL-ku ra-Z?
When was the last time?	Когда был последний раз?	kug-DA bil pus-L-YED-nee raz?
New	Новое	NO-vu-ye
Old	Старое	STA-ru-ye

CONTEXT

Did you...?	NA (see below)	NA (see below)
fall	Вы упали?	vi oo-PA-lee?
trip	Вы споткнулись?	vi stuk-NOO-lees?
faint	Вы упали в обморок?	vi oo-PA-lee v OB-mu-ruk?
twist	Вы подвернулись?	vi pud-v-yer-NOO-lees?
get hit	Вы ударились?	vi oo-da-REE-lees?
get burned	Вы получили ожоги?	vi pu-loo-CHEE-lee u-ZHO-gee?
get assaulted	На вас напали?	na vas na-PA-lee?
get bitten (human/dog/cat/insect)	Вас кто-то укусил?	vas oo-koo-SEE-lu sh-TO-tu?

PAST MEDICAL HISTORY

Take medication?	Вы принимаете медикаменты?	pree-nee-MA-ye-t-ye mee-dee-ka-M-YEN-ti?
(aspirin/ antibiotics)	(аспирин/ антибиотики)	as-pee-REE-n / an-tee-bee-O-tee-kee)
Do you have (See also Medical Problem List)...	Есть ли у вас...	YES-t lee oo vas...

(cont.)

allergies	алергии	a-L-YER-gee-ye
medical problems	медицинские проблемы	mee-dee-TSEEN-skee-ye prub-L-YE-mi
Do you have problems of the…(see Body Parts List)	Проблемы с…	prub-L-YE-mi s…

SURGICAL HISTORY

Have you had surgery?	Вас оперировали?	vas u-pee-REE-ru-va-lee?
Surgery on/"to remove"…(see Body Parts List)	Операция на…	u-pee-RA-tsee-ya

SOCIAL HISTORY

Smoke?	Курите?	KOO-ree-t-ye?
Drink?	Пьёте алкоголь?	P-YO-t-ye al-ku-GOL?
Take drugs?	Пользуетесь наркотиками?	POL-zoo-yee-tees nar-KO-ti-ka-mi?
Recent travel?	Путешествовали ли вы недавно?	poo-tee-SH-EST-vu-va-lee nee-DAF-no?
Are you sexually active?	Вы сексуально активны?	vi seek-soo-AL-nu ak-TIV-ni?
Do you use condoms?	Вы используете презервативы?	vi ees-POL-zoo-yee-tee pree-zer-va-TEE-vi?
Homosexual	Вы гомосексуалист?	vi gu-mu-s-yek-soo-a-LEEST?

SYSTEMS REVIEW

Do you have…	Есть ли у вас…	YES-t lee oo vas…

GENERAL

Fever	Жар	zhar
Chills	Озноб	uz-NOP

Weight loss	Потеря веса?	pu-t-yer-YA v-YE-sa?
Fatigue	Усталость	oo-STA-lust
Sick contact	Контакты с больными людьми?	kun-TAK-T s BOL-ni-mi l-yood-MI?
HEENT		
Sore throat	Боль в горле?	BOL v GOR-l-ye
Runny nose	Насморк	NAS-murk
Nosebleed	Кровотечение из носа	kru-vu-t-ye-CH-YE-nee-ye eez NO-sa
Ear pain	Ушная боль	OOSH-na-ya bol
Ear ringing	Звонит в ушах?	z-VO-neet voo-SHAKH?
Decreased hearing	Плохой слух	oo-m-yen-SH-YE-nee s-lookh
EYE		
Eye pain	Глазная боль	G-LAZ-nu-yu BOL?
Blurry vision	Неясное зрение	nee-YAS-nu-ye z-R-YE-nee-ye
Diplopia	Двойное зрение	d-VOY-nu-ye z-R-YE-nee-ye
Foreign body sensation	Чувство постороннего тела	CHOOV-st-vo pu-stu-RO-nee-vu T-YE-lu
Contact lenses	Контактные линзы	kun-TAKT-nee-ye LEEN-zi
CARDIAC		
Chest pain	Боль в груди	bol v groo-DEE
Palpitations	Учащённое сердцебиение	oo-chash-CH-YON-nu-ye s-yerd-ts-ye-bee-YE-nee-ye
Orthopnea	Трудно дышать, когда лежите?	TROOD-nu DI-shat, kug-DA lee-ZHI-t-ye?

(cont.)

Dyspnea on exertion	Трудно дышать, когда ходите?	TROOD-nu DI-shat, kug-DA KHO=dee-t-ye?
Fainting (syncope)	Обморок	OB-mu-ruk
Leg swelling	Опухание ног	u-poo-KHA-nee-ye nok
How many pillows?	Сколько подушек нужно, чтобы дышать нормально?	SKOL-ku pu-DOO-shek NOOZH-nu, sh-TO-bi DI-shat nur-MAL-nu?
PULMONARY		
Trouble breathing	Трудно дышать?	TROOD-nu di-shat?
SOB	Одышка / Нехватает воздуха?	u-DISH-ka / nee-kh-VA-ta-yeet VOZ-doo-kha?
Cough	Кашель	KA-shel
Sputum	Мокрота	mu-kru-TA
Pain on inspiration	Боль при вдохе	BOL pree v-DOKH-ye
Hemoptysis	Кровавый кашель	kru-VA-vee KA-shel
GI		
Abdominal pain	Боль в животе	bol v zhi-vo-T-YE
Nausea	Тошнота	tush-nu-TA
Vomiting	Рвота	r-VO-ta
Vomiting blood	Рвота с кровью	r-VO-ta s KROV-yoo
Coffee ground emesis	Рвота, похожая на кофейную гущу	r-VO-ta, pu-KHO-zha-ya na ku-F-YEY-noo-yoo GOOSH-choo
Anorexia	Отсутствие аппетита	ut-SOOT-st-vee-ye ap-p-ye-TEE-ta
Diarrhea	Понос	pu-NOS

Difficulty swallowing	Трудности при глотании	TROOD-nus-tee pree glu-TA-nee-yee
BRBPR	Кровотечение алой кровью из прямой кишки	kru-vu-t-ye-CH-YEN-ye A-luy KROV-yoo eez p-R-YA-muy KEESH-kee
Melena	Дегтеобразный стул	d-YEG-t-ye-u-BRAZ-nee stool
Pain after eating	Боли после еды	BO-lee POS-l-ye YE-di
Worms	Глисты	glees-TI
Constipation	Запор	ZA-pur

GU

Painful urination	Болезненное мочеиспускание	bul-yez-N-YE-nu-ye mu-ch-ye-ees-poos-KA-nee-ye
Urgent urination	срочное мочеиспускание/ нетерпение	s-KROCH-nu-ye mu-ch-ye-ees-poos-KA-nee-ye / nee-t-yer-P-YE-nee-ye
Frequent urination	Частое мочеиспускание	CHAST-nu-ye mu-ch-ye-ees-poos-KA-nee-ye
Bloody urination	Кровь в моче	KROV v mu-CH-YE
Discharge: vaginal/penile	Выделения из влагалища (vaginal)/ выделения из пениса (penile)	vi-d-yel-YE-nee-ya eez v-la-GA-lee-sha (vaginal) / vi-dee-L-YE-nee-ya eez p-YE-nee-sa (penile)

PSYCH

Anxiety	Тревога	tree-VO-ga
Depression	Депрессия	dee-pr-YES-see-ya
Suicidal thoughts	Мысли о самоубийстве	MIS-lee O sa-mu-oo-BEEST-v-ye

(cont.)

Homicidal thoughts	Желание кого-то убить	zhe-LA-nee-ye ku-VO tu oo-BEET
Medication overdose	Передозировка лекарства	pee-ree-do-zee-ROV-ka lee-KARS-t-vu
Hear voices	Слуховые галлюцинации	sloo-KHO-vee-ye gal-l-yoo-tsee-NA-tsee-yee
NEURO		
Headache	Головная боль	gu-luv-NA-ya BOL
Worst headache of life	Самая сильная головная боль в жизни	SA-ma-ya SEEL-na-ya gu-lu-VA-ya bol v ZHIZ-nee
Weakness	Слабость	SLA-bust
Dizzy	Головокружение	gu-lu-vu-kroo-ZHE-nee-ye
What is your name?	Как вас зовут?	kak vas zu-VOOT?
Where are we?	Где мы находимся?	g-D-YE mi na-KHO-deem-s-ya?
What is the year/month/date?	Какой сейчас год/ месяц/ какая сегодня дата?	ka-KOY see-CHAS GO-D /M-YE-syats / ka-KA-ya see-VO-D-n-ya DA-ta?
Bowel dysfunction	Кишечные расстройства	ki-SHECH-ni-ye r as-STROY-st-va
Bladder dysfunction	Расстройство мочевого пузыря	ras-STROY-st-vu mu-CH-YE-vu-vu poo-zir-YA
Photophobia	Чувствительность к свету	choov-st-VEE-t-yel-nust K s-V-YE-too
Tingling/ numbness	Ощущение покалывания или онемения	u-shoo-SHE-nee-ye pa-KA-li-va-nee-yu ee-lee u-nee-M-YE-nee-ya

Decreased strength in... (See Body Parts List)	Ослабление....	u-slub-L-YE-nee-ye...
Seizure	Конвульсия	kun-VOOL-see-yu
Difficulty walking	Трудности при ходьбе	TROOD-nu-stee pree khud-B-YE
Difficulty speaking	Затруднённая речь	za-trood-N-YON-nu-yu r-YECH
Spinning (vertigo)	Головокружение	gu-lu-vu-kroozh-N-YE-nee-ye
Confusion	Растерянность	rus-t-yer-YAN-nust
MISC		
Lump	Вздутие	v-z-DOO-tee-ye
Itching	Зуд	ZOOD
Bruising	Ушиб	oo-SHEEP
Rash	Сыпь	sip
Swelling	Отечность	u-T-YOCH-nust
Jaundice (yellow skin)	Желтуха	zhel-TOO-kha
GYNECOLOGIC		
Vaginal bleeding	Вагинальные кровотечения	va-gee-NAL-ni-ye kru-vu-t-ye-CH-YE-nee-yu
Heavy	Сильные	SEEL-ni-ye
Irregular	нерегулярные	nee-ree-gool-YAR-ni-ye
Absent	Отсутствующее	ut-soot-st-VOO-yoosh-chee-ye
Vaginal discharge	Вагинальные выделения	va-gee-NAL-ni-ye vi-d-ye-L-YE-nee-yu

(cont.)

Pelvic pain	Тазовая боль	TAZ-u-va-ya bol
Rape	Изнасилование	eez-na-SEEL-u-va-nee-ye
Pain with intercourse	Боль при половом контакте	BOL pree pu-lu-VOM kun-TAK-t-ye
Contraceptive	Противозачаточное средство	pru-tee-vu-za-CHA-tuch-nu-ye s-R-YED-st-vu

OBSTETRIC

Are you pregnant?	Вы беременны?	vi bee-R-YO-m-ye-ni?
LMP how many days ago?	Сколько дней назад была последняя менструация?	SKOL-ku d-N-YEY na-ZAD BI-la pus-L-YED-na-ya meen-stroo-A-tsee-ya?
Times pregnant?	Сколько раз были вы беременны?	SKOL-ku raz BI-lee vi bee-R-YO-m-ye-ni?
Times delivered?	Слько раз рожали?	SKOL-ku raz ru-ZHA-lee?
Miscarriage	Выкидыш	VI-kee-dish
Abortion	Аборт	a-BORT
Fluid leakage	Утечка жидкости	oo-T-YECH-ka ZHID-kus-tee
Contraction	Сокращение/ Родовая схватка	su-kra-SH-YON-nee-ye/ru-du-VA-yu s-kh-VAT-ku
Fetal movement	Движение плода	d-vee-ZHE-nee-ye PLO-da

TRAUMA

How many hours ago did you eat last?	Сколько часов назад вы ели в последний раз?	SKOL-ku chu-SOF na-ZAD vi YE-lee v pus-L-YED-nee ras?
Lost consciousness?	Вы теряли сознание?	vi t-yer-YA-lee suz-NA-nee-ye?

Russian — Русский язык

Tetanus within 5 years?	Делали ли вам за последние пять лет прививку от столбняка?	D-YE-l-u-lee lee vam za pus-L-YED-nee-ye p-YAT L-YET pree-VEEV-koo ot stol-b-N-YA-ku?
PEDIATRIC		
How old?	Каков возраст ребенка? Сколько дней (days) / месяцев (months) / лет (years)?	ku-KOF VOZ-rust r-ye-B-YON-ka? SKOL-ku d-N-YEY (days) / M-YES-ya-tsef (months) / L-YET (years)
Vaccines up to date?	Все ли прививки сделаны?	f-S-YE lee pree-VEEV-kee s-D-YE-la-ni?
Urinating normally	Мочится нормально	MO-cheet-su nur-MAL-nu
Taking liquids	Пьёт жидкости?	P-YOT ZHID-kus-tee
Increased crying	Плачет больше обычного	PLA-cheet BOL-she u-BICH-nu-vu
Ingestion	Проглотил что-то (ядовитое)	pru-glu-TEEL sh-TU-tu (yu-du-VEE-tu-ye)
Foreign body	Инородное тело	ee-nu-ROD-nu-ye T-YE-lu
Premature	Преждевременные роды	PR-YEZH-deev-r-ye-M-YEN-nee-ye RO-di
Birth complications	Осложнения при родах	us-luzh-N-YE-nee-yu pree RO-dakh
PHYSICAL EXAM//INSTRUCTION		
Sit down (please)	Садитесь (пожалуйста)	sa-DEE-t-yes (pu-ZHA-looy-sta)
Lie down	Лягте	L-YAG-t-ye
Come here	Подойдите	pu-duy-DEE-t-ye

(cont.)

Relax	Расслабтесь	ra-SLAB-t-yes
Don't move	Не двигайтесь	nee d-VEE-gay-t-yes
Open your mouth	Откройте рот	ut-KROY-t-ye rot
Say "ahh"	Скажите «Ааа»	ska-ZHEE-t-ye "Aaa"
Swallow	Сглотните	glut-NEE-t-ye
Breath deeply	Вдыхайте глубоко	v-di-KHAY-t-ye gloo-bu-KO
Hold your breath	Задержите дыхание	za-d-yer-ZHI-t-ye di-KHA-nee-ye
Cough	Кашляйте	KASH-l-yay-t-ye
Push	Толкайте	Tul-KAY-t-ye
Pull	Тяните	t-ya-NEE-t-ye
Follow my finger	Следите глазами за моим пальцем	sl-ye-DEE-t-ye gla-ZA-mee za mu-YEEM PAL-tseem
Close your eyes	Закройте глаза	za-KROY-t-ye gla-ZA
Smile	Улыбнитесь	oo-lib-NEE-t-yes
Can you feel this?	Чувствуете это?	CHOOV-st-voo-ye-t-ye E-tu?
Copy this (movement)	Сделайте так.	s-D-YE-lay-t-ye TAK
I am going to put a finger in your rectum	Я сейчас вставлю палец в прямую кишку	ya see-CHAS v-stav-L-YOO PA-leets b P-R-YA-moo-yoo KEESH-koo
I am going to examine your vagina	Я осмотрю влагалище	ya us-MOT-r-yoo v-la-GA-leesh-ch-ye
REASSESSMENT		
Do you feel better?	Вы себя лучше чувствуете?	vi seeb-YA LOO-che CHOOST-voo-ye-t-ye?

Do you feel worse?	Вы себя хуже чувствуете?	vi see-B-YA KHOO-zhe CHOOV-st-voo-ye-t-ye?

PATIENT WORDS

I hurt	Мне болит	m-n-YE bu-LEET
Help!	Помогите	pu-mu-GEE-t-ye
Bathroom	Туалет	too-a-L-YET
Food	Пища / еда	PEE-sha / yee-DA
Water	Вода	vu-DA

PROCEDURES & CONSENT

You need...	Вам требуется...	vam TR-YE-boo-yet-s-ya...
Injection	Инъекция/ укол	een-YEK-tsee-ya / OO-kul
Stiches	Швы	sh-VI
Cast	Гипс	GEEP-s
Crutches	Костыли	Kus-TI-lee
Perform surgery on the... (See Body Parts List)	Оперировать на....	u-p-yee-REE-ro-vat na...
The risks are...	Риски...	REES-kee
Bleeding	кровотечение	kru-vu-tu-CH-YE-nee-ye
Infection	Инфекция	een-F-YEK-tsee-ya
Scar	шрам	sh-RAM
Repeat procedure	Повторить процедуру	Puv-tu-REET pru-tsee-DOO-roo
Iodine	Йод	yod
Damage to your... (See Body Parts List)	Повреждение...	puv-r-yezh-D-YE-nee-ye...

(cont.)

Sign here	Подпышите здесь	pud-pi-SHEE-t-ye z-D-YES
TESTS		
X-ray	Рентген	R-YENT-geen
C.A.T. Scan	Компьютерная томография (К.Т.)	kum-P-YOO-teer-na-ya tu-mu-GRA-fee-ya (ka-te)
Ultrasound	Ультразвук	ool-tra-z-VOOK
Catheterization/ bladder catheter	Катетризация /введение катетера в мочевой пузырь	ku-t-yer-ee-ZA-tsee-yu / v-v-ye-D-YE-nee-ye ka-T-YE-tee-ra v mu-chee-VOY POO-zeer
Colonoscopy (from below)/ Endoscopy (from above)	Колоноскопия	ku-lu-nus-KO-pee-ya
Endoscopy	Эндоскопия	en-dus-KO-pee-ya
END OF LIFE		
Do you want us to…	Хотите ли вы, чтобы мы…	khu-TEE-t-ye lee VI sh-TO-bi mi…
Perform CPR	сделали сердечно-легочную реанимацию (СЛР)	s-D-YE-la-le s-yer-D-YECH-nu-lee-GOCH-noo-yoo ree-a-nee-MA-tsee-yoo (es-el-er)
Defibrillate	сделали дефибриляцию	s-D-YE-la-le dee-fee-bree-LA-tsee-yoo?
Intubate	ввели дыхательную трубку в гортань	v-V-YE-lee di-kha-t-YEL-noo-yoo TROOB-koo v gur-TAN
He/she is dead	Он умер (he)/ Она умерла (she)	on OO-m-yer (he)/ u-NA OO-m-yer-la
We did all we could	Мы сделали всё, что могли	mi s-D-YE-la-lee f-S-YO, sh-TO mug-LEE

Russian—Русский язык

DISCHARGE		
You have…(See Medical Prob List)	У вас есть...	oo vas YES-t...
He/she is going to stay in the hospital	Он / Она остаётся в больнице	on (he)/ u-NA (she) u-sta-YOT-s-ya v BOL-nee-ts-ye
Take "X" pills "Y" times a day for "Z" days	Принимайте "X" таблетки "Y" раз в день в течение "Z" дней	pree-nee-MAY-t-ye "X" tab-L-YET-kee "Y" raz v d-YEN v t-ye-CH-YE-nee-ye "Z" d-N-YEY
Pills	Таблетки	tab-L-YET-kee
Antibiotics	Антибиотики	an-tee-bee-O-tee-kee
Before/after meals	Перед едой / после еды	P-YE-reed ye-DOY / POS-l-ye ye-DI
Return to the ER if…	Вернитесь в пункт неотложной помощи, если...	veer-NEE-t-yes v POON-k-t nee-ut-LO-ZH-nuy PO-mu-shee, YES-lee
Follow up at "X" on "Y"	Пойти в "X" в "Y"	puy-TEE V "X" v "Y"
You're welcome	Пожалуйста	pu-ZHA-looy-sta
Goodbye	до свидания	du-s-vee-DA-nee-yu
MEDICAL PROBS		
AIDS/HIV	СПИД / ВИЧ	speed / veech (ve-ee-che)
Anemia	Анемия	a-NYE-mee-ya
Arrhythmia	Аритмия	a-REET-mee-ya
Arthritis	Артрит	ar-TREET
Asthma	Астма	AST-ma
Bronchitis	Бронхит	brun-KHEET
Cancer	Рак	rak

(cont.)

Cirrhosis	Цирроз	tseer-ROZ
Cholesterol	Холестерин	khu-lees-tee-REEN
Cold	Насморк	NAS-murk
Constipation	Запор	ZA-pur
Cyst	Киста	kees-TA
Diabetes	Диабет	dee-a-B-YET
Dialysis	Диализ	dee-A-leez
Diverticulitis	Дивертикулит	dee-veer-tee-koo-LEET
Emphysema	Эмфизема	em-fee-Z-YE-ma
Fibroids	Фиброма	fee-BRO-ma
Fracture	Перелом	pee-ree-LOM
Flu	Грипп	greep
Gallstones	Жёлчный камень	ZHOL-ch-nee KA-meen
Gastritis/GERD	Гастрит	gas-TREET
Hepatitis	Гепатит	gee-pa-TEET
Heart attack	Инфаркт / Сердечный припадок	een-FAR-K-T / seer-D-YECH-nee pree-pa-DOK
Heart disease	Болезнь сердца (инфаркт) / Порок сердца	bu-L-YEZ-n S-YERD-tsu (een-FAR-kt) / pu-ROK S-YER-d-tsu
Heart failure	Сердечная недостаточность Разрыв сердца	s-yer-D-YECH-nu-yu nee-dus-tu-TOCH-nust / raz-RIV S-YERD-tsu
Hypertension	Гипертония	gee-peer-TO-nee-ya
Indigestion	Несварение / Расстройство желудка	nees-vur-YE-nee-ye / ras-STROY-st-vu zhi-LOOD-ku

Kidney stone	Почечный камень	PO-ch-yech-niy KA-m-yen
Lupus	Волчанка	vul-CHAN-ka
Migraine	Мигрень	Mee-GR-YEN
Murmur	Шум в сердце	shoom v S-YERD-ts-ye
Pacemaker	Стимулятор сердца	stee-moo-L-YA-tur S-YERD-tsa
Pneumonia	Воспаление лёгких	vus-pa-L-YE-nee-ye L-YOG-keekh
Seizures	Конвульсии / Эпилептический припадок	kun-VOOL-see-ee / e-pee-leep-TEE-chees-kee pree-pa-DOK
STD	Венерическая болезнь	vee-nee-REE-chees-ka-ya bu-L-YEZ-n
Stroke	Удар / инсульт	OO-dar / een-SOOLT
Ulcer	Язва	YAZ-va
Ulcerative colitis	Язвенный колит	yaz-V-YEN-nee ku-LEET
UTI	Инфекция мочевых путей	een-F-YEK-tsee-ya mu-chee-VIKH poo-T-YEY
BODY PARTS		
Abdomen	Живот	zhee-VOT
Ankle	Лодыжка	lu-DIZH-ka
Appendix	Аппендикс	ap-P-YEN-deeks
Arm	Рука	roo-KA
Artery	Артерия	ar-T-YE-ree-ya
Back	Спина	spee-NA

(cont.)

Bladder	Мочевой пузырь	mu-chee-VOY POO-zir
Blood	Кровь	KROF
Bone	Кость	kost
Brain	Мозг	MOZ-k
Breast	грудь	grood
Calf	Икра	eek-RA
Chest	Грудь	grood
Chin	Подбородок	pud-bu-RO-duk
Ear	Ухо	OO-khu
Elbow	Локоть	LO-kut
Eye	Глаз	glaz
Face	Лицо	lee-TSO
Finger	Палец	PA-leets
Foot	Нога	nu-GA
Hand	Рука	roo-KA
Head	Голова	gu-lu-VA
Heart	Сердце	S-YERD-tse
Gallbladder	Жёлчный пузырь	ZHOL-ch-nee POO-zir
Jaw	Челюсть	chee-L-YOOST
Joint	Сустав	soos-TAF
Kidney	Почка	POCH-ka
Knee	Колено	ku-L-YE-nu
Leg	Нога	nu-GA
Liver	Печень	pee-CHEN
Mouth	Рот	rot
Muscle	Мышца	MISH-tsa

Russian—Русский язык

Neck	Шея	SHE-ya
Nerve	Нерв	nerv
Nose	Нос	nos
Ovary	Яичник	ya-EECH-neek
Pancreas	Поджелучная железа	pud-zhe-LOOCH-na-ya zhe-lee-ZA
Penis	мужской половой член	moozh-KOY pu-lu-VOY ch-L-YEN
Prostate	Предстательная железа	preed-STA-teel-na-ya zhe-lee-ZA
Rectum	Прямая кишка	P-R-YA-ma-ya KEESH-ka
Rib	Ребро	reeb-RO
Shoulder	Плечо	PL-YE-chu
Skin	Кожа	KO-zha
Spleen	Селезёнка	see-lee-Z-YON-ka
Spine	Спина/Хребет	spee-NA / kh-ree-B-YET
Stomach	Желудок	zhe-LOO-duk
Teeth	Зубы	ZOO-bi
Testicle	Яичко	YA-eech-ku
Throat	Горло	GOR-lu
Thyroid	Щитовидная железа	sh-chee-tu-VEED-na-ya zhe-lee-ZA
Toe	палец ноги	PA-leets NO-gee
Tonsils	Миндалины	meen-DA-lee-ni
Tongue	Язык	ya-ZIK
Uterus	Матка	MAT-ka
Vagina	влагалище	v-la-GA-leesh-che

Vein	Вена	V-YE-na
Wrist	Запястье	za-P-YAS-t-ye

NUMBERS

How many (times)?	Сколько раз?	SKOL-ku RAS?
0	Ноль	Nool
1	Один	u-DEEN
2	Два	d-VA
3	Три	tree
4	Четыре	chee-TI-ree
5	Пять	p-YAT
6	Шесть	Shest
7	Семь	s-YEM
8	Восемь	VO-s-yeem
9	Девять	D-YEV-yat
10	Десять	D-YES-yat
11	Одиннадцать	u-DIN-nad-ts-yat
20	Двадцать	d-VAD-ts-yat
30	Тридцать	TREED-ts-yat
40	Сорок	SO-ruk
50	Пятьдесят	P-YAT-dees-yat
60	Шестьдесят	SHEST-dees-yat
70	Семьдесят	S-YEM-dees-yat
80	Восемьдесят	VOS-yem-dees-yat
90	Девяносто	dee-v-ya-NO-stu
100	Сто	STO

Spanish—Español

WORD/PHRASE	TRANSLATION	ENGLISH PRONUNCIATION
Spanish	Español	es-pan-YOL
INTRODUCTION		
Hello	Hola	O-la
I am a doctor / nurse	Soy doctor (masc) / doctora (fem) / enfermero (masc) / enfermera (fem)	soy dok-TOR/a / en-fer-MER-o/a
What is your name?	¿Cómo se llama?	KO-mo se YA-ma?
Who is your doctor?	¿Quién es su doctor?	kee-EN es soo dok-TOR?
How old are you?	¿Cuántos años tiene?	K-WAN-tos AN-yos tee-E-ne?
Birthdate?	¿Fecha de nacimiento?	FE-cha de na-see-mee-EN-to?
Telephone number?	¿Número de teléfono?	NOO-me-ro de te-LE-fo-no?
Address?	¿Dirección?	dee-rek-see-ON?
Social security number?	¿Número de Seguro Social?	NOO-mer-o de se-GOO-ro so-see-AL?
Insurance?	¿Seguro?	se-GOO-ro
BASICS		
Do you understand?	¿Me entiende Usted?	me en-tee-EN-de oo-STED?
Yes	Sí	see
No	No	no
Please	Por favor	por fa-VOR
Thank you	Gracias	GRA-see-as
Sorry	Lo siento	lo see-EN-to

(cont.)

I don't understand	No entiendo	no en-tee-EN-do
Repeat	Repita	re-PEE-ta
Speak slowly	Hable lentamente	AB-le len-ta-MEN-te
Answer "yes" or "no"	Conteste "sí" o "no"	con-TES-te 'see' o 'no'
Here	Aquí	a-KEE
This	Esto	ES-to
It's alright (consoling)	Está bien	es-TA b-YEN
I'll be right back	Ya vengo	ya VENG-o

GENERAL

What's wrong?	¿Qué tiene?	KE tee-E-ne
Pain	Dolor	do-LOR
Do you have pain?	¿Tiene dolor?	tee-E-ne do-LOR?
Does the pain radiate?	¿Le corre el dolor?	le KORR-e el do-LOR?
Where (show me)	¿Dónde? (muéstreme)	DON-de? (M-WES-tre-me)
Gone now	¿Ya se le quitó?	ya se le kee-TO?
Still present	¿Lo tiene ahora mismo?	LO tee-E-ne a-O-ra MEES-mo?
Sudden/gradual onset	de repente / poco a poco	de re-PEN-te / PO-ko a PO-ko
What bothers you the most?	¿Qué es lo que le molesta más?	KE es lo ke le mo-LES-ta mas?
Why did you come today?	¿Por qué vino hoy?	por-KE VEE-no oy?

QUALITY

If '0' is no pain and 10 is maximum pain, what number do you have now?	Si el número cero es ningún dolor y diez es dolor máximo, ¿qué número tiene en este momento?	si el NOO-me-ro SE-ro es neen-GOON do-LOR EE dee-ES es do-LOR MAK-see-mo, ke NOO-mero tee-E-ne en ES-te MO-men-to?

Burning	¿Le arde?	le AR-de?
Constant	Constante	kon-STAN-te
Dull	Embotado	em-bo-TA-do
Intermittent	Va y viene	va ee vee-E-ne
Pressure	Presión	pre-see-ON
Severe	Fuerte	F-WER-te
Sharp/prickly pains	Dolores agudos/ punzantes	do-LO-res a-GOO-do/ poon-SAN-tes
Throbbing	Pulsante	pool-SAN-te
ASSOCIATED SYMPTOMS		
Onset during… (before/after)	¿Qué hacía Usted cuando se le comenzó esto? (antes / después?)	KE a-SEE-a oo-STED K-WAN-do se le ko-men-SO ES-to (AN-tes / des-P-WES?)
Worse (with…)	Está peor (con)	es-TA pe-OR (con)
Better (with…)	Está mejor (con)	es-TA me-khor (con)
Cough	Tos	tos
Deep breath	Al respirar profundamente	AL res-pee-RAR pro-foon-da-MEN-te
Emotional upset	Trastorno emocional	tras-TOR-no e-mo-see-o-NAL
Food	Comida	ko-MEE-da
Movement	Movimiento	mo-vee-mee-EN-to
Nothing	Nada	NA-da
Positioning	En alguna posición	en al-GOO-na po-see-see-ON
Rest	Al descansar	AL des-kan-SAR
Walking	Al caminar	AL ka-mee-NAR

(cont.)

TIME COURSE		
For how long?	¿Duránte cuánto tiempo?	doo-RAN-te K-WAN-to tee-EM-po?
Today	Hoy	oy
Yesterday	Ayer	a-YER
How many...	¿Cuántos / as...?	K-WAN-tos / tas?
Months/weeks/days/hours/seconds	Meses / semanas / días / horas / segundos	ME-ses / se-MA-nas / DEE-as / O-ras / se-GOON-dos
Still present?	¿Todavía tiene?	to-da-VEE-a tee-E-ne?
Gone now?	¿Ya se le quitó?	ya se le kee-TO?
How long did it last? (See Numbers List)	¿Cuánto tiempo duró?	K-WAN-to tee-EM-po doo-RO?
Have you had this before?	¿Ha tenido esto antes?	A te-NEE-do ES-to AN-tes?
How many times?	¿Cuantas veces?	K-WAN-tas VE-ses
When was the last time?	¿Cuándo fue la última vez?	KWAN-do fwe la OOL-tee-ma ves?
New	Nuevo	nu-E-vo
Old	Viejo	vee-E-kho
CONTEXT		
Did you...?	¿Es que Usted..?	es ke oo-STED...?
fall	se cayó	se ka-YO?
trip	se tropezó	se tro-pe-SO?
faint	se desmayó	se des-ma-YO?
twist	se torció algo	se tor-see-O AL-go?
get hit	se golpió	se gol-pee-O?
get burned	se quemó	se ke-MO?

get assaulted	fue asaltado/a (masc / fem)	F-WE a-sal-TA-do/a?
get bitten (human/dog/cat/insect)	fue mordido/a (masc / fem)	F-WE mor-DEE-do/a?
PAST MEDICAL HISTORY		
Take medication?	¿Toma medicamentos?	TO-ma me-dee-ka-MEN-tos?
(aspirin/antibiotics)	aspirina / antibióticos	as-pee-REE-na / an-tee-bee-O-tee-kos?
Do you have (See also Medical Problem List)...	¿Tiene...	tee-E-ne..?
allergies	alergias	a-LER-khee-as?
medical problems	problemas médicos	prob-LE-mas ME-dee-kos
Do you have problems of the... (see Body Parts List)	¿Tiene problemas de...	tee-E-ne prob-LE-mas de...
SURGICAL HISTORY		
Have you had surgery?	¿Ha tenido cirugía?	A te-NEE-do see-roo-KHEE-a?
Surgery on/"to remove"...(see Body Parts List)	Cirugía de...	see-roo-KHEE-a de...
SOCIAL HISTORY		
Smoke?	¿Fuma?	FOO-ma?
Drink?	¿Toma?	TO-ma?
Take drugs?	¿Usa drogas?	OO-sa DRO-gas?
Recent travel?	¿Ha viajado recien?	a vee-a-KHA-do re-see-EN?
Are you sexually active?	¿Tiene relaciones sexuales?	tee-E-ne re-la-see-O-nes sek-soo-A-les?

(cont.)

Do you use condoms?	¿Usa preservativos?	OO-sa pre-ser-va-TEE-vos?
Homosexual	Homosexual	o-mo-sek-soo-AL

SYSTEMS REVIEW

Do you have...	¿Tiene..?	tee-E-ne..?

GENERAL

Fever	Fiebre	fee-E-vre?
Chills	Escalofríos	es-ka-lo-FREE-os
Weight loss	Pérdida de peso	PER-dee-da de PE-so
Fatigue	Cansancio	kan-SAN-see-o
Sick contact	Contacto con enfermos	kon-TAK-to con en-FER-mos

HEENT

Sore throat	Dolor de la garganta	do-LOR de la gar-GAN-ta
Runny nose	Flujo de la nariz	FLOO-kho de la na-REES
Nosebleed	Sangre de la nariz	SAN-gre de la na-REES
Ear pain	Dolor del oído	do-LOR del-o-EE-do
Ear ringing	Zumbido	soom-BEE-do
Decreased hearing	Disminución del oído / ensordece Usted?	dees-mee-noo-see-ON del o-EE-do / en-sor-DE-se oo-STED?

EYE

Eye pain	Dolor del ojo	do-LOR del-O-kho
Blurry vision	Vista borrosa	VEE-sta bo-RRO-sa
Diplopia	Vista doble	VEE-sta DO-ble
Foreign body sensation	Sensación de que hay algo en el ojo	sen-sa-see-ON de ke ay AL-go en el O-kho
Contact lenses	Lentes de contacto	LEN-tes de kon-TAK-to

CARDIAC		
Chest pain	Dolor del pecho	do-LOR del PE-cho
Palpitations	Palpitaciones	pal-pee-ta-see-O-nes
Orthopnea	¿Sensación de que se ahoga cuando se acuesta plano?	sen-sa-see-ON de ke se a-O-ga K-WAN-do se a-K-WES-ta PLA-no
Dyspnea on exertion	¿Falta de aire cuando camina?	FAL-ta de AY-re K-WAN-do ka-MEE-na
Fainting (syncope)	Desmayo	des-MA-yo
Leg swelling	Piernas hinchadas	pee-ER-nas een-CHA-das
How many pillows?	¿Cuántas almohadas necesita para domir?	K-WAN-tas al-mo-A-das ne-se-SEE-ta PA-ra dor-MEER?
PULMONARY		
Trouble breathing	¿Le cuesta respirar?	le K-WES-ta res-pee-RAR?
SOB	Falta de aire	FAL-ta de AY-re
Cough	Tos	TOS
Sputum	Flema	FLE-ma
Pain on inspiration	Dolor cuando inspira	do-LOR K-WAN-do een-SPEE-ra
Hemoptysis	Tos con sangre	TOS kon SAN-gre
GI		
Abdominal pain	Dolor del estómago	do-LOR del es-TO-ma-go
Nausea	Náusea	NAU-se-a
Vomiting	Vómito	VO-mee-to
Vomiting blood	Vómito con sangre	VO-mee-to kon SAN-gre
Coffee ground emesis	Vómito que parece poso de café	VO-mee-to ke pa-RE-se PO-so de ka-FE

(cont.)

Anorexia	Falta de hambre	FAL-ta de AM-bre
Diarrhea	Diarrea	dee-a-RRE-a
Difficulty swallowing	Dificultad para tragar	dee-fee-kool-TAD PA-ra tra-GAR
BRBPR	Sangre roja del recto	SAN-gre RO-kha del REK-to
Melena	Excremento que parece brea negra	es-kre-MEN-to ke pa-RE-se BRE-a NE-gra
Pain after eating	Dolor después de comer	do-LOR des-P-WES de ko-MER
Worms	Parásitos / Lombríces	pa-RA-see-tos / lom-BREE-ses
Constipation	Estreñimiento	es-tre-n-yee-mee-EN-to
GU		
Painful urination	Dolor cuando orina	do-LOR K-WAN-do o-REE-na
Urgent urination	Necesita orinar urgentemente	ne-se-SEE-ta o-ree-NAR oor-khen-te-MEN-te
Frequent urination	Necesita orinar frecuentemente	ne-se-SEE-ta o-ree-NAR fre-KWEN-te-MEN-te
Bloody urination	Sangre en la orina	SAN-gre en la o-REE-na
Discharge: vaginal/penile	Descarga de: la vagina / del pene	des-KAR-ga de: la VA-khee-na / del PE-ne
PSYCH		
Anxiety	Ansiedad	an-see-e-DAD
Depression	Depresión	de-pre-see-ON
Suicidal thoughts	¿Ha pensado en dañarse?	a pen-SA-do en dan-YAR-se?
Homicidal thoughts	¿Ha pensado en dañar a culaquier otro?	a pen-SA-do en dan-YAR a k-wal-K-YER O-tro?
Medication overdose	Sobredosis de medicación	SO-bre-DO-sees de me-dee-ka-see-ON

Hear voices	¿Oye voces de personas que no están ahí?	O-ye VO-ses de per-SO-nas ke no es-TAN a-EE?
NEURO		
Headache	Dolor de cabeza	do-LOR de ka-BE-sa
Worst headache of life	¿Dolor de cabeza más fuerte de la vida?	do-LOR de ka-BE-sa MAS F-WER-te de la VEE-da?
Weakness	Debilidad	de-bee-lee-DAD
Dizzy	Mareos	ma-RE-os
What is your name?	¿Cómo se llama?	KO-mo se YA-ma?
Where are we?	¿Donde estamos?	DON-de es-TA-mos?
What is the year/month/date?	¿Cuál es la fecha hoy?	k-wal es la FE-cha oy?
Bowel dysfunction	Problemas al defecar	prob-LE-mas al de-fe-KAR
Bladder dysfunction	Problemas al orinar	prob-LE-mas al o-ree-NAR
Photophobia	¿Le irrita la luz?	le EE-rree-ta la luz?
Tingling/numbness	Hormigueos / Entumecimiento	or-mee-GE-os / en-too-me-see-mee-EN-to
Decreased strength in…(See Body Parts List)	Debilidad de…	de-bee-lee-DAD
Seizure	Convulsiones	kon-vool-see-O-nes
Difficulty walking	Dificultad para caminar	dee-fee-kool-TAD PA-ra ka-mee-NAR
Difficulty speaking	Dificultad para hablar	dee-fee-kool-TAD PA-ra a-BLAR
Spinning (vertigo)	¿Se siente que el cuarto se gira?	se see-EN-te ke el K-WAR-to se KHEE-ra?
Confusion	¿Se siente confuso/a?	se see-EN-te kon-FOO-so/a?

(cont.)

MISC		
Lump	Un bulto / Una bola	un BOOL-ta/OO-na BOL-a
Itching	Comezón	ko-me-SON
Bruising	Moretón	mo-re-TON
Rash	Erupción / roncha	e-roop-see-ON / RON-cha
Swelling	Hinchazón	een-cha-SON
Jaundice (yellow skin)	Ictericia (piel amarilla)	eek-te-REE-see-a/pee-EL a-ma-REE-ya
GYNECOLOGIC		
Vaginal bleeding	¿Le sale sangre de la vagina?	le SA-le SAN-gre de la VA-khee-na?
Heavy	Con exceso	kon ek-SE-so
Irregular	Irregular	ee-re-gu-LAR
Absent	¿Tiene reglas?	tee-E-ne REG-las?
Vaginal discharge	Descarga de la vagina	des-KAR-ga de la VA-khee-na
Pelvic pain	Dolor pélvico	do-LOR PEL-vee-ko
Rape	Violación	vee-o-la-see-ON
Pain with intercourse	Dolor con relaciones sexuales	do-LOR kon re-la-see-O-nes sek-soo-A-les
Contraceptive	Anticonceptivo	an-tee-kon-sep-TEE-vo
OBSTETRIC		
Are you pregnant?	¿Está embarazada?	es-TA em-ba-ra-SA-da?
LMP how many days ago?	¿Cuándo fue la última regla?	K-WAN-do f-we la OOL-tee-ma REG-la?
Times pregnant?	¿Cuántos embarazos ha tenido?	K-WAN-tos em-ba-RA-sos a te-NEE-do?
Times delivered?	¿Cuántos nacieron?	K-WAN-tos na-see-E-ron?
Miscarriage	Aborto involuntario	a-BOR-to een-vo-loon-TA-ree-o

Abortion	Aborto	a-BOR-to
Fluid leakage	¿Le sale líquido?	le SA-le LEE-kee-do?
Contraction	Contracción	kon-trak-see-ON
Fetal movement	Movimiento del bebé	mo-vee-mee-EN-to del be-BE
TRAUMA		
How many hours ago did you eat last?	¿Cuándo fue la última vez que comió?	K-WAN-do f-we la OOL-tee-ma ves ke ko-mee-O?
Lost consciousness?	¿Perdió el conocimiento?	per-dee-O el ko-no-see-mee-EN-to?
Tetanus within 5 years?	¿La vacuna contra el tétano dentro de 5 años?	la va-KOO-na KON-tra el TE-ta-no DEN-tro de SEEN-ko AN-yos?
PEDIATRIC		
How old?	¿Cuántos años tiene?	K-WAN-tos AN-yos tee-E-ne?
Vaccines up to date?	¿Las vacunas están corrientes?	las va-KOO-nas es-TAN ko-ree-EN-tes?
Urinating normally	¿Orina normalmente?	o-REE-na nor-mal-MEN-te?
Taking liquids	¿Está tomando líquidos?	es-TA to-MAN-do LEE-kee-dos?
Increased crying	¿Llora más que lo normal?	YO-ra mas ke lo nor-MAL?
Ingestion	¿Podría haber tomado algo tóxico?	po-DREE-a a-BER to-MA-do AL-go TOK-see-ko?
Foreign body	¿Podría tener algún objeto adentro?	po-DREE-a te-NER al-GOON ob-KHE-to a-DEN-tro?
Premature	Prematuro	pre-ma-TOO-ro

(cont.)

| Birth complications | Complicaciones con el parto | kom-plee-ka-see-O-nes kon el PAR-to |

PHYSICAL EXAM/INSTRUCTION

Sit down (please)	Siéntese (por favor)	see-EN-te-se (por fa-VOR)
Lie down	Acuéstese	a-K-WES-te-se
Come here	Venga	VEN-ga
Relax	Relájese	re-LA-khe-se
Don't move	No se mueva	no se M-WE-va
Open your mouth	Abra la boca	A-bra la BO-ka
Say "ahh"	Diga "ahh"	DEE-ga "A"
Swallow	Trague	TRA-ge
Breath deeply	Respire profundamente	res-PEE-re pro-foon-da-MEN-te
Hold your breath	Mantenga la respiración	man-TEN-ga la res-pee-ra-see-ON
Cough	Tosa	TO-sa
Push	Empuje	em-POO-khe
Pull	Jale	KHA-le
Follow my finger	Siga el dedo	SEE-ga el DE-do
Close your eyes	Cierre los ojos	see-E-re los O-khos
Smile	Sonría	son-REE-a
Can you feel this?	¿Siente esto?	see-EN-te ES-to?
Copy this (movement)	Haga lo que yo hago	A-ga lo ke yo A-go
I am going to put a finger in your rectum	Voy a poner un dedo en el recto	voy a po-NER un DE-do en el REK-to
I am going to examine your vagina	Voy a examinar la vagina	voy a ek-sa-mee-NAR la VA-khee-na

REASSESSMENT		
Do you feel better?	¿Se siente mejor?	se see-EN-te me-KHOR?
Do you feel worse?	¿Se siente peor?	se see-EN-te pe-OR?
PATIENT WORDS		
I hurt	Me duele	me D-WE-le
Help!	¡Ayuda!	a-YOO-da!
Bathroom	Baño	BAN-yo
Food	Comida	ko-MEE-da
Water	Agua	A-g-wa
PROCEDURES & CONSENT		
You need…	Necesita…	ne-se-SEE-ta…
Injection	Una inyección	OO-na een-yek-see-ON
Stiches	Puntadas	poon-TA-das
Cast	Yeso	YE-so
Crutches	Muletas	moo-LE-tas
Perform surgery on the… (See Body Part List)	Hacer cirugía sobre…	a-SER see-roo-KHEE-a SO-bre…
The risks are…	Los riesgos son…	los ree-ES-gos son…
Bleeding	Sangrar	san-GRAR
Infection	Infectarse	een-fek-TAR-se
Scar	Dejar cicatríz	de-KHAR see-ka-TREES
Repeat procedure	Repitir la procedura	re-pee-TEER la pro-se-DOO-ra
Iodine	Yodo	YO-do
Damage to your… (See Body Parts List)	Daño a…	DAN-yo
Sign here	Firme aquí	FEER-me a-KEE

(cont.)

TESTS		
X-ray	Radiografía / placas	ra-dee-o-gra-FEE-a / PLA-kas
C.A.T. Scan	Radiografía CT (placas computerizadas)	ra-dee-o-gra-FEE-a se-te / PLA-kas kom-poo-ter-ee-SA-das
Ultrasound	Ultrasonido	ool-tra-so-NEE-do
Catheterization/ bladder catheter	Cateterización / sonda	ka-te-te-ree-sa-see-ON / SON-da
Colonoscopy (from below)/Endoscopy (from above)	Colonoscopía (por abajo)/Endoscopía (por boca)	ko-lo-nos-ko-PEE-a (por a-BA-kho)/en-dos-ko-PEE-a (por BO-ka)
Endoscopy	Endoscopía	en-do-sco-PEE-a
END OF LIFE		
Do you want us to...	¿Quiere que hagamos...	kee-E-re ke a-GA-mos...
Perform CPR	compresiones / resucitación cardiopulmonar	kom-pre-see-O-nes / re-soo-see-ta-see-YON kar-dee-o-pool-mo-NAR
Defibrillate	desfibrilación/darle choque eléctrico	des-fee-bree-la-see-ON/ dar-le CHO-ke e-LEK-tree-ko
Intubate	intubar / ponerle tubo en el pasaje de aire	een-too-BAR / po-NER-le TOO-bo en el pa-SA-khe de AY-re
He/she is dead	Él / ella está muerto/a	el/EY-ya es-TA m-WER-to/a
We did all we could	Hicimos todo lo que pudimos	ee-SEE-mos TO-do lo ke poo-DEE-mos
DISCHARGE		
You have...(See Medical Prob List)	Tiene...	tee-E-ne...
He/she is going to stay in the hospital	Él / ella se va a quedar en el hospital	el / EY-ya se va a ke-DAR en el os-pee-TAL

Take "X" pills "Y" times a day for "Z" days	Tome "X" píldoras "Y" veces al día por "Z" días	TO-me "X" PEEL-do-ras "Y" ve-ses al DEE-a por "Z" DEE-as
Pills	Píldoras / pastillas	PEEL-do-ras / pas-TEE-yas
Antibiotics	Antibióticos	an-tee-bee-O-tee-kos
Before/after meals	Antes / después de la comida	AN-tes / des P-WES de la ko-MEE-da
Return to the ER if…	Vuelva a la Urgencia si…	V-WEL-va a la oor-KHEN-see-a see…
Follow up at "X" on "Y"	Vaya a "X" el "Y"	VA-ya a "X" el "Y"
You're welcome	No hay de qué	no ay de KE
Goodbye	¡Adiós!	a-dee-OS
MEDICAL PROBS		
AIDS/HIV	SIDA	SEE-da
Anemia	Anemia	a-NE-mee-a
Arrhythmia	Arritmia	a-RREET-mee-a
Arthritis	Artritis	ar-TREE-tees
Asthma	Asma	AS-ma
Bronchitis	Bronquitis	bron-KEE-tees
Cancer	Cáncer	KAN-ser
Cirrhosis	Cirrosis del higado	see-RRO-sees del EE-ga-do
Cholesterol	Colesterol (alto)	ko-les-te-ROL (AL-to)
Cold	Un resfrío / resfriado / catarro	res-FREE-o / res-free-A-do / ka-TA-rro
Constipation	Estreñimiento	es-tre-n-yee-mee-EN-to
Cyst	Quiste	KEES-te
Diabetes	Diabetes	dee-a-BE-tes

(cont.)

Dialysis	Diálisis	dee-A-lee-sees
Diverticulitis	Diverticulitis	dee-ver-eei-koo-LEE-tees
Emphysema	Enfisema	en-fee-SE-ma
Fibroids	Fibroma uterino (de la matríz)	fee-BRO-ma oo-te-REE-no (de la ma-TREES)
Fracture	Fractura	frak-TOO-ra
Flu	Gripe/gripa	GREE-pe/GREE-pa
Gallstones	Cálculos biliares (piedras en la vesícula)	KA-koo-los bee-lee-A-res (pee-E-dras en la ve-SEE-koo-la)
Gastritis/GERD	Gastritis (reflujo / acidez)	gas-TREE-tees (re-FLOO-kho / a-see-DES)
Hepatitis	Hepatitis	e-pa-TEE-tees
Heart attack	Ataque de corazón	a-TA-ke de ko-ra-SON
Heart disease	Enfermedad de corazón	en-fer-me-DAD de ko-ra-SON
Heart failure	Insuficiencia cardiaca	een-su-fee-see-EN-see-a kar-dee-A-ka
Hypertension	Hipertensión (presión alta)	ee-per-ten-see-ON (pre-see-ON AL-ta)
Indigestion	Indigestión	een-dee-khes-tee-ON
Kidney stone	Cálculo renal (piedra en el riñón)	KAL-koo-lo re-NAL (pee-E-dra en el reen-YON)
Lupus	Lupus	Loo-poos
Migraine	Migraña	mee-GRAN-ya
Murmur	Soplo	SO-plo
Pacemaker	Marcapasos	mar-ka-PA-sos
Pneumonia	Neumonía	ne-oo-mo-NEE-a
Seizures	Convulsiones	kon-vool-see-O-nes
STD	Enfermedad sexual	en-fer-me-DAD sek-soo-AL

Stroke	Derrame cerebral / ataque cerebral	de-RRA-me se-re-BRAL / a-TA-ke se-re-BRAL
Ulcer	Úlcera	OOL-se-ra
Ulcerative colitis	Colitis ulcerosa	ko-LEE-tees ool-se-RO-sa
UTI	Cistitis (infección de la vejiga)	sees-TEE-tees (een-fek-see-ON de la ve-KHEE-ga)

BODY PARTS

Abdomen	El abdomen	el AB-do-men
Ankle	El tobillo	el to-BEE-yo
Appendix	El apéndice	el a-PEN-dee-se
Arm	El brazo	el BRA-so
Artery	La arteria	la ar-TE-ree-a
Back	La espalda	la es-PAL-da
Bladder	La vejiga	la ve-KHEE-ga
Blood	La sangre	la SANG-re
Bone	El hueso	el WE-so
Brain	El cerebro	el se-RE-bro
Breast	El pecho / el seno (of a woman)	el PE-cho / el SE-no
Calf	La pantorrilla	la pan-to-REE-a
Chest	El pecho	el PE-cho
Chin	El mentón	el men-TON
Ear	La oreja	la o-RE-kha
Elbow	El codo	el KO-do
Eye	El ojo	el O-kho
Face	La cara	la KA-ra
Finger	El dedo	el DE-do

(cont.)

Foot	El pie	el pee-E
Hand	La mano	la MA-no
Head	La cabeza	la ka-BE-sa
Heart	El corazón	el ko-ra-SON
Gallbladder	La vesícula (biliar)	la ve-SEE-koo-la
Jaw	La mandíbula	la man-DEE-boo-la
Joint	La articulación	la ar-tee-koo-la-see-ON
Kidney	El riñon	el reen-YON
Knee	La rodilla	la ro-DEE-ya
Leg	La pierna	la pee-ER-na
Liver	El hígado	el EE-ga-do
Mouth	La boca	la BO-ka
Muscle	El músculo	el MOOS-koo-lo
Neck	El cuello	el koo-EY-yo
Nerve	El nervio	el NER-vee-o
Nose	La nariz	la na-REES
Ovary	El ovario	el o-VA-ree-o
Pancreas	El páncreas	el PAN-kre-as
Penis	El pene	el PE-ne
Prostate	La próstata	la PRO-sta-ta
Rectum	El recto	el REK-to
Rib	La costilla	la kos-TEE-ya
Shoulder	El hombro	el OM-bro
Skin	La piel	la pee-EL
Spleen	El bazo	el BA-so
Spine	La columna (vertebral)	la ko-LOOM-na
Stomach	El estómago	el es-TO-ma-go

Teeth	Los dientes	los dee-EN-tes
Testicle	El testículo	el tes-TEE-koo-lo
Throat	La garganta	la gar-GAN-ta
Thyroid	El tiroides	el tee-ROY-des
Toe	El dedo del pie	el DE-do del pee-E
Tonsils	Las amígdalas	las a-MEEG-da-las
Tongue	La lengua	la LENG-wa
Uterus	El útero / la matriz	el OO-te-ro/la ma-TREES
Vagina	La vagina	la VA-khee-na
Vein	La vena	la VE-na
Wrist	La muñeca	la moon-YE-ka
NUMBERS		
How many (times)?	¿Cuantas veces?	K-WAN-tas VE-ses
0	Cero	SE-ro
1	Uno	OO-no
2	Dos	dos
3	Tres	tres
4	Cuatro	K-WA-tro
5	Cinco	SEEN-ko
6	Seis	seys
7	Siete	see-E-te
8	Ocho	O-cho
9	Nueve	noo-E-ve
10	Diez	dee-ES
11	Once	ON-se
20	veinte	VEYN-te

(cont.)

30	treinta	TREYN-ta
40	cuarenta	kwa-REN-ta
50	cincuenta	seen-KWEN-ta
60	sesenta	se-SEN-ta
70	setenta	se-TEN-ta
80	ochenta	o-CHEN-ta
90	noventa	no-VEN-ta
100	cien	see-EN

Tagalog (Filipino)—Tagalog

WORD/PHRASE	TRANSLATION	ENGLISH PRONUNCIATION
Tagalog	Tagalog	ta-GA-log
INTRODUCTION & REGISTRATION		
Hello	kamusta	ka-moos-TA
I am doctor / nurse *(add your name)*	ako si doktor / a-nars *(add your name)*	a-KO see dok-TOR / A-NARS *(add your name)*
What is your name?	ano ang pangalan mo?	a-NO ANG pa-NGA-lan mo?
Who is your doctor?	sino ang doktor mo?	SEE-no ANG dok-TOR mo?
How old are you?	Ilang taon ka na?	ee-LANG tah-ON ka-NA?
Birthdate?	kapanganakan?	ka-PA-nga-NA-kan?
Telephone number?	numero ng telepono?	NOO-me-ro NANG te-LE-po-no?
Address?	tirahan?	tee-RA-han?
Social security number?	numero ng social security?	NOO-me-ro NANG SOO-shal seek-YOO-ree-tee?
Insurance?	insurance?	een-SHOO-rans?
BASICS		
Do you understand?	naiintindihan mo?	na-ee-EEN-teen-dee-HAN mo?
Yes	oo	O-o
No	hindi	HEEN-dee
Please	paki	pa-KEE
Thank you	salamat	sa-LA-mat
Sorry	sori	SO-ree
I don't understand	hindi ko naiintindihan	HEEN-dee ko na-ee-EEN-teen-dee-HAN

(cont.)

Repeat	paki-ulit	pa-KEE OO-leet
Speak slowly	magsalita ng mabagal	mag-sa-lee-TA nang ma-BA-gal
Answer "yes" or "no"	sagot ng "oo" o "hindi"	sa-GOT nang "O-o" o "HEEN-dee"
Here	dito	DEE-to
This	ito	ee-TO
It's alright (consoling)	sige lang	see-ge lang
I'll be right back	babalik ako	ba-ba-LEEK a-KO

GENERAL

What's wrong?	ano ang problema?	a-NO ANG prob-LE-ma?
Pain	masakit	ma-sa-KEET?
Do you have pain?	may masakit?	may ma-sa-KEET?
Does the pain radiate?	kumakalat ba ang sakit	KOO-ma-ka-lat BA ang sa-KEET?
Where (show me)	saan ang masakit?	sa-AN ang ma-sa-KEET?
Gone now	wala na?	wa-LA na?
Still present	mayroon pa?	may-roo-ON pa?
Sudden/gradual onset	bigla/unti-unti sumakit?	beeg-LA/oon-TEE oon-TEE soo-ma-KEET?
What bothers you the most?	saan pinakamasakit?	sa-AN pee-na-KA-ma-sa-KEET?
Why did you come today?	bakit pumunta ka dito ngayon?	ba-KEET poo-moon-TA ka DEE-to nga-YON?

QUALITY

If "0" is no pain and 10 is maximum pain, what number do you have now?	kung "cero" walang sakit at sampu pinakamasakit, anong numero mayron ka?	koong "SE-ro" wa-LANG sa-KEET at sam-POO pee-na-KA-ma-sa-KEET, a-nong NOO-me-ro may-ron KA?
Burning	mahapdi	ma-HAP-dee

Constant	palagi	pa-LA-gee
Dull	medyo masakit	MED-yo ma-sa-KEET
Intermittent	nawawala at bumabalik	na-WA-wa-la at bu-Ma-ba-leek
Pressure	parang dinaganan	PA-rang dee-na-ga-NAN
Severe	pinakamasakit	pee-na-KA-ma-sa-KEET
Sharp/prickly pains	parang tinusok	PA-rang tee-NOO-sok
Throbbing	parang may pulso	PA-rang may pool-SO
ASSOCIATED SYMPTOMS		
Onset during… (before/after)	Umpisa ng sakit/ katapusan ng sakit	OOM-pee-sa nang sa-KEET / ka-TA-poo-SAN nang sa-KEET
Worse (with…)	mas masakit (kapag…)	mas ma-sa-KEET ka-PAG…
Better (with…)	mas mabuti (kapag…)	mas ma-BOO-tee ka-PAG…
Cough	ubo	oo-BO
Deep breath	huminga ng malalim	hoo-mee-NGA-nang ma-LA-leem
Emotional upset	nasaktan ang damdamin	na-sak-TAN ang dam-DA-meen
Food	pagkain	pag-KA-een
Movement	gumalaw	goo-ma-LAU
Nothing	wala	wa-LA
Positioning	posisyon	po-sees-YON
Rest	nagpahinga	NAG-pa-hee-NGA
Walking	naglakad	NAG-la-KAD
TIME COURSE		
For how long?	gaano katagal	ga-A-no ka-ta-GAL

(cont.)

Today	ngayon	nga-YON
Yesterday	kahapon	ka-HA-pon
How many...	ilan...	ee-LAN...
Months/weeks/days/hours/seconds	buwan/lingo/araw/oras/segundo	boo-WAN/leeng-GO/A-rau/O-ras/se-GOON-do
Still present?	mayroon pa ngayon?	may-roo-ON pa nga-YON?
Gone now?	wala na?	wa-LA na?
How long did it last? (See Numbers)	gaano katagal sumakit?	ga-A-no ka-ta-GAL soo-ma-KEET?
Have you had this before?	nangyari na ito noon?	nang-YA-ree na ee-TO noo-ON?
How many times?	ilang beses?	ee-LANG BE-ses?
When was the last time?	kailan huling nangyari?	ka-ee-LAN hoo-LEENG nang-YA-ree?
New	bago	BA-go
Old	luma	LOO-ma?

CONTEXT

Did you...?	ikaw ba ay...	ee-KAU ba ay...
fall	nahulog	na-HOO-log
trip	nadapa	na-da-PA
faint	hinimatay	hee-nee-ma-TAY
twist	natapilok	na-ta-pee-LOK
get hit	tinamaan	TEE-na-MA-an
get burned	napaso	na-PA-so
get assaulted	nabugbog	na-boog-BOG?
get bitten (human/dog/cat/insect)	nakagat	na-ka-GAT

PAST MEDICAL HISTORY

Take medication?	umiinom ka ba ng gamot?	oo-mee-ee-NOM ka ba nang ga-MOT?

(aspirin/antibiotics)	aspirina/antibiotico	as-pee-REE-na/ an-TEE-bee-O-tee-co
Do you have (See also Medical Problem List)…	mayroon ka bang…	may-roo-ON ka BANG…
allergies	alerhiya	a-ler-HEE-ya
medical problems	problema sa kalusugan	prob-LE-ma SA ka-loo-SOO-gan
Do you have problems of the… (see Body Parts List)	mayroon ka bang problema sa…	may-roo-ON ka BANG prob-LE-ma SA…
SURGICAL HISTORY		
Have you had surgery?	sumailalim ka na ba ng operasyon?	soo-ma-ee-LA-leem ka na BA nang o-pe-ras-YON?
Surgery on/"to remove"…(see Body Parts List)	operasyon sa…	o-pe-ras-YON SA…
SOCIAL HISTORY		
Smoke?	naninigarilyo?	na-nee-nee-ga-REEL-yo?
Drink?	umiinom?	oo-mee-ee-NOM?
Take drugs?	nagdu-droga?	nag-doo-DRO-ga?
Recent travel?	kagagaling mo lang sa biyahe?	ka-ga-GA-leeng mo LANG sa bee-YA-he?
Are you sexually active?	nakikipagtalik ka?	na-kee-kee-pag-TA-leek ka?
Do you use condoms?	gumagamit ka ba ng kondom?	goo-ma-GA-meet ka BA nang KON-dom?
Homosexual	may gusto sa pareho mong kasarian?	may gus-TO sa pa-RE-ho mong ka-sa-REE-an?
SYSTEMS REVIEW		
Do you have…	mayroon ka bang…	may-ro-ON ka bang….

(cont.)

GENERAL		
Fever	lagnat	lag-NAT
Chills	pan-lalamig	pan-LA-la-meeg
Weight loss	pagkawala ng timbang	pag-ka-wa-LA NANG teem-BANG
Fatigue	matinding pagod	ma-teen-DEENG PA-gud
Sick contact	kinahawaan	kee-NA-ha-WA-an
HEENT		
Sore throat	sakit sa lalamunan	sa-KEET sa la-la-MOO-nan
Runny nose	sipon	SEE-pon
Nosebleed	dugo sa ilong	doo-GO sa ee-LONG
Ear pain	sakit sa tenga	sa-KEET sa TE-nga
Ear ringing	ingay sa pandinig	EE-ngay sa pan-dee-NEEG
Decreased hearing	pang-hihina sa pandinig	pang-hee-HEE-na sa pan-dee-NEEG
EYE		
Eye pain	sakit sa mata	sa-KEET sa ma-TA
Blurry vision	panlalabo sa paningin	pan-la-LA-bo sa pa-nee-NGEEN
Diplopia	doble sa paningin	DOB-le sa pa-nee-NGEEN
Foreign body sensation	puwing sa mata	poo-WEENG sa ma-TA
Contact lenses	kontak lens	KON-tak lens
CARDIAC		
Chest pain	sakit sa dibdib	sa-KEET sa deeb-DEEB
Palpitations	mabilis na tibok ng puso	ma-bee-LEES na tee-BOK nang POO-so

Orthopnea	hirap sa paghinga kapag nakahiga	HEE-rap sa pag-hee-NGA ka-PAG na-ka-hee-GA
Dyspnea on exertion	pagsikip ng hininga kapag pumwersa	pag-see-KEEP NANG hee-nee-NGA ka-PAG poom-WER-sa
Fainting (syncope)	pagkahimatay	pag-ka-HEE-ma-tay
Leg swelling	pamamaga sa binte	pa-ma-ma-GA sa BEEN-te
How many pillows?	ilang unan ang gamit mo sa pagtulog?	EE-lang OO-nan ang GA-meet mo SA pag-TOO-log
PULMONARY		
Trouble breathing	hirap sa paghinga	HEE-rap sa pag-hee-NGA
SOB	kinakapos sa paghinga	kee-na-ka-POS sa pag-hee-NGA
Cough	ubo	oo-BO
Sputum	plema	PLE-ma
Pain on inspiration	sakit kapag huminga ng malalim	sa-KEET ka-PAG hoo-mee-NGA nang ma-LA-leem
Hemoptysis	dugo sa plema	doo-GO sa PLE-ma
GI		
Abdominal pain	sakit sa tiyan	sa-KEET sa tee-YAN
Nausea	nasusuka	na-SOO-soo-KA
Vomiting	pagsusuka	PAG-soo-soo-KA
Vomiting blood	dugo sa suka	doo-GO sa SOO-ka
Coffee ground emesis	nagsusuka nang parang sapa ng kape	nag-SOO-soo-KA nang PA-rang koo-lay nang ka-PE
Anorexia	anoreksia	a-no-REK-sya
Diarrhea	pagtatae	pag-TA-ta-EE

(cont.)

Difficulty swallowing	hirap sa paglunok	HEE-rap SA pag-loo-NOK
BRBPR	sariwang dugo sa pwet	sa-REE-wang du-GO sa poo-WET
Melena	maitim na tae	ma-ee-TEEM na TA-e
Pain after eating	sakit sa tiyan pagkatapos kumain	sa-KEET sa tee-YAN pag-ka-TA-pos koo-MA-een
Worms	bulate	boo-LA-te
Constipation	matigas na tae	ma-tee-GAS na TA-e
GU		
Painful urination	sakit sa pag-ihi	sa-KEET sa pag-EE-hee
Urgent urination	kailangang kailangang umihi	ka-ee-LA-ngang ka-ee-LA-ngang u-MEE-hee
Frequent urination	madalas na pag-ihi	ma-da-LAS na pag-EE-hee
Bloody urination	dugo sa ihi	doo-GO sa EE-hee
Discharge: vaginal/penile	tulo sa ari?	TOO-lo sa A-ree
PSYCH		
Anxiety	nerbiyos	ner-be-YOS
Depression	depresyon	de-pres-YON
Suicidal thoughts	balak magpakamatay?	ba-LAK mag-pa-KA-ma-TAY?
Homicidal thoughts	balak pumatay?	ba-LAK poo-ma-TAY?
Medication overdose	nasobrahan sa gamot	na-SO-bra-HAN sa ga-MOT
Hear voices	naririnig na mga boses	na-ree-ree-NEEG na mga BO-ses
NEURO		
Headache	sakit sa ulo	sa-KEET sa OO-lo

Worst headache of life	pinaka grabeng sakit sa ulo	pee-na-KA GRA-beng sa-KEET sa OO-lo
Weakness	panghihina	pang-hee-HEE-na
Dizzy	panghihilo	pang-hee-HEE-lo
What is your name?	ano ang pangalan mo?	a-NO ang pa-NGA-lan mo?
Where are we?	nasaan tayo?	NA-sa-an TA-yo?
What is the year/month/date?	ano ang taon / buwan / araw?	a-NO ang ta-ON / BOO-wan / A-rau?
Bowel dysfunction	problema sa pagtae	prob-LE-ma sa pag-TA-e
Bladder dysfunction	problema sa pantug	prob-LE-ma sa PAN-tog
Photophobia	sensitibo sa ilaw	sen-see-TEE-bo sa EE-lau
Tingling/numbness	pakiramdam may tumutusok /pagkawala ng pakiramdam	pa-kee-ram-DAM may-too-mooTOO-sok/ pag-ka-wa-LA nang pa-kee-RAM-dam
Decreased strength in…(See Body Part List)	panghihina	pang-hee-HEE-na
Seizure	kombulsion	kom-BOL-si-on
Difficulty walking	hirap sa paglalakad	HEE-rap sa PAG-la-la-kad
Difficulty speaking	hirap sa pagsasalita	HEE-rap sa pag-SA-sa-lee-TA
Spinning (vertigo)	pagkahilo	pag-ka-HEE-lo
Confusion	pagkalito	pag-ka-lee-TO
MISC		
Lump	bukol	BOO-kol
Itching	pangangati	pa-NGA-nga-tee
Bruising	pasa	pa-SA

(cont.)

Rash	butlig	BOOT-lig
Swelling	pamamaga	pa-ma-ma-GA
Jaundice (yellow skin)	paninilaw ng balat	pa-nee-nee-LAU ng ba-LAT

GYNECOLOGIC

Vaginal bleeding	pagdurugo sa ari	pag-DOO-roo-go sa A-ree
Heavy	matindi	ma-teen-DEE
Irregular	lumalaktaw	loo-MA-lak-TAU
Absent	kawalan	KA-wa-lan
Vaginal discharge	tulo sa ari	TOO-lo sa A-ree
Pelvic pain	sakit sa balakang	sa-KEET sa ba-la-KANG
Rape	ginahasa	gee-na-HA-sa
Pain with intercourse	sakit sa pagtatalik	sa-KEET sa pag-ta-TA-leek
Contraceptive	kontrasepsion	KON-tra-sep-SYON

OBSTETRIC

Are you pregnant?	buntis ka ba?	boon-TEES ka BA?
LMP how many days ago?	huling regla	hoo-LEENG REG-la
Times pregnant?	ilang beses nagbuntis?	ee-LANG BE-ses nag-boon-TEES?
Times delivered?	ilang beses nanganak?	ee-LANG BE-ses na-nga-NAK?
Miscarriage	ilang beses nakunan?	ee-LANG BE-ses na-KOO-nan?
Abortion	ilang beses nagpalaglag?	ee-LANG BE-ses nag-pa-lag-LAG?
Fluid leakage	basag na tubig	ba-SAG na TOO-beeg
Contraction	kontraksion	kon-trak-SYON
Fetal movement	paggalaw ng sangol	pag-ga-LAU ng sang-GOL

TRAUMA		
How many hours ago did you eat last?	kailan ka huling kumain	ka-ee-LAN ka hoo-LEENG koo-MA-een?
Lost consciousness?	nawalan ng malay	na-wa-LAN nang MA-lay?
Tetanus within 5 years?	bakuna sa tetano sa nakaraang limang taon	ba-KOO-na sa TE-ta-no sa na-KA-ra-ANG lee-MANG ta-ON?
PEDIATRIC		
How old?	ilang taon?	ee-LANG ta-ON?
Vaccines up to date?	kompletong bakuna	kom-PLE-tong ba-KOO-na
Urinating normally	umiihi ng maayos	oo-mee-EE-hee nang ma-A-yos
Taking liquids	umiinom ng maayos	oo-mee-ee-NOM nang ma-A-yos
Increased crying	mas madalas na pag-iyak	mas ma-da-LAS na pag-ee-YAK
Ingestion	lumunok	loo-mo-NOK
Foreign body	kakaibang bagay	ka-ka-ee-BANG BA-gay
Premature	napaagang panganganak	NA-pa-A-gang pa-nga-nga-NAK
Birth complications	kumplikasion sa panganganak	koom-plee-ka-SION sa pa-nga-nga-NAK
PHYSICAL EXAM/INSTRUCTION		
Sit down (please)	maupo ka	ma-oo-PO ka
Lie down	humiga ka	hoo-mee-GA ka
Come here	halika	ha-LEE-ka
Relax	kalmado lang	kal-MA-do lang
Don't move	huwag gagalaw	hoo-WAG GA-ga-lau

(cont.)

Open your mouth	buksan ang bunganga	book-SAN ang boo-NGA-nga
Say "ahh"	mag "ahh"	mag "ahh"
Swallow	lunok	loo-NOK
Breath deeply	huminga ng malalim	hoo-mee-NGA NANG ma-LA-leem
Hold your breath	itigil ang paghinga	ee-TEE-geel ang pag-hee-NGA
Cough	ubo	oo-BO
Push	itulak	ee-TOO-lak
Pull	hilahin	hee-LA-heen
Follow my finger	sundan ang daliri ko	soon-DAN ang da-LEE-ree ko
Close your eyes	isarado ang mata	ee-sa-RA-do ang ma-TA
Smile	ngiti	ngee-TEE
Can you feel this?	nararamdaman mo ito	na-RA-ram-da-MAN mo ee-TO
Copy this (movement)	gayahin mo ito	ga-YA-heen mo ee-TO
I am going to put a finger in your rectum	ipapasok ko ang aking daliri sa pwet mo	ee-pa-PA-sok ko ang A-keeng da-LEE-re sa poo-wet mo
I am going to examine your vagina	eksaminin ko ang ari mo	ek-sa-MEE-neen ko ang A-ree mo
REASSESSMENT		
Do you feel better?	bumuti ba pakiramdam mo	boo-MOO-tee ba pa-kee-RAM-dam mo
Do you feel worse?	lumala ba ang pakiramdam mo	loo-ma-LA ba ang pa-kee-RAM-dam mo
PATIENT WORDS		
I hurt	may masakit sa akin	may ma-sa-KEET sa A-keen

Help!	tulungan	TOO-loong-ngan
Bathroom	banyo	BAN-yo
Food	pagkain	pag-KA-een
Water	tubig	TOO-beeg
PROCEDURES & CONSENT		
You need...	kailangan mo ng...	ka-ee-LA-ngan mo nang....
Injection	iniksion	ee-neek-SYON
Stiches	tahi	ta-HEE
Cast	semiento	SEE-mee-YEN-to
Crutches	saklay	sak-LAY
Perform surgery on the... (See Body Part List)	operasion sa....	o-pe-ra-SYON sa....
The risks are...	peligro na kaakibat...	pe-LEE-gro na ka-a-KEE-bat...
Bleeding	pagdurugo	pag-DOO-roo-go
Infection	impeksion	eem-pek-SYON
Scar	peklat	PEK-lat
Repeat procedure	pag-ulit sa operasyon	pag-OO-leet sa o-pe-ra-SYON
Iodine	iodina	ee-yo-DEE-na
Damage to your... (See Body Part List)	pinsala	peen-SA-la
Sign here	pumirma dito	poo-meer-MA DEE-to
TESTS		
X-ray	x-ray	EX-rey
C.A.T. Scan	ct eskan	see-tee-es-KAN
Ultrasound	ultrasound	OOL-tra-SOUND

(cont.)

Catheterization/ bladder catheter	tubo sa pantug	TOO-bo sa pan-TOOG
Colonoscopy (from below)/Endoscopy (from above)	kamera sa bituka	KA-me-ra sa bee-TOO-ka
Endoscopy	kamera sa tiyan	KA-me-ra sa TEE-yan

END OF LIFE

Do you want us to...	gusto nyo ba kaming....	gus-TO nyo ba ka-MEENG...
Perform CPR	e-CPR kayo	e-SEE-PEE-ER ka-YO
Defibrillate	e-defibrillate kayo	e-de-fee-bree-LEYT ka-YO
Intubate	magpasok ng tubo para kayo makahinga	mag-PA-sok nang TOO-bo PA-ra ka-YO ma-ka-hee-NGA
He/she is dead	(ikinalulungkot ko) pumanaw na sya	(ee-kee-na-loo-loong-KOT ko) poo-MA-nau na see-YA
We did all we could	ginawa namin lahat ng aming makakaya	gee-na-WA NA-meen la-HAT nang A-meeng ma-ka-KA-ya

DISCHARGE

You have...(See Medical Prob List)	mayroon...	may-ro-ON...
He/she is going to stay in the hospital	kailangan syang manatili sa ospital	ka-ee-LA-ngan see-YANG ma-na-TEE-lee sa os-pee-TAL
Take "X" pills "Y" times a day for "Z" days	uminom ng "X" tableta "Y" beses sa isang araw sa loob ng "Z" araw	oo-mee-NOM nang "X" tab-LE-ta "Y" BE-ses sa ee-SANG A-rau sa lo-OB nang "Z" A-ra
Pills	tableta / pilduras	tab-LE-ta / peel-DOO-ras
Antibiotics	antibiotik	an-tee-bay-O-teek
Before/after meals	bago / pagkatapos kumain	BA-go / pag-ka-TA-pos koo-MA-een

Return to the ER if...	bumalik sa ER kapag...	boo-ma-LEEK sa E-R ka-PAG...
Follow up at "X" on "Y"	bumalik sa "X" sa "Y"	boo-ma-LEEK sa "X" sa "Y"
You're welcome	walang anuman	wa-LANG A-noo man
Goodbye	paalam	pa-A-lam
MEDICAL PROBS		
AIDS/HIV	AIDS/HIV	AIDS/HIV
Anemia	anemya	a-NEM-ya
Arrhythmia	aritmia	a-REET-mee-ya
Arthritis	artritis	ar-TREE-tees
Asthma	hika	HEE-ka
Bronchitis	bronkitis	bron-KEE-tees
Cancer	kanser	KAN-ser
Cirrhosis	mga peklat sa atay	ma-NGA PEK-lat sa a-TAY
Cholesterol	kolesterol	ko-LES-te-rol
Cold	sipon	see-PON
Constipation	tibi	TEE-bee
Cyst	bukol	BOO-kol
Diabetes	diyabetis	dee-ya-BE-tees
Dialysis	diyalisis	dee-YA-lee-SEES
Diverticulitis	namamaga na bituka	na-MA-ma-GA na bee-TOO-ka
Emphysema	empisema	em-pee-SE-ma
Fibroids	bukol sa bahay bata	BOO-kol sa BA-hay BA-ta
Fracture	bali sa buto	BA-lee sa boo-TO
Flu	trangkaso	trang-KA-so
Gallstones	bato sa apdo	ba-TO sa ap-DO

(cont.)

Gastritis/GERD	namamaga na sikmura	na-MA-ma-GA na seek-MOO-ra
Hepatitis	hepatitis	he-pa-TEE-tees
Heart attack	atake sa puso	a-TA-kee sa POO-so
Heart disease	sakit sa puso	sa-KEET sa POO-so
Heart failure	mahinang puso	ma-HEE-nang POO-so
Hypertension	"high blood" / alta presyon	hay BLUD / AL-ta pre-see-ON
Indigestion	hindi natunawan	heen-DEE na-too-NA-wan
Kidney stone	sakit sa bato	sa-KEET sa ba-TO
Lupus	lupus	LOO-poos
Migraine	migrayn	MAY-greyn
Murmur	abnormal na tunog sa puso	ab-nor-MAL na too-NOG sa POO-so
Pacemaker	"pacemaker" para regular ang tibok ng puso	"pacemaker" PA-ra re-goo-LAR ang tee-BOK nang POO-so
Pneumonia	pulmonya	pool-mon-YA
Seizures	kombolsyon	kom-bol-see-ON
STD	tulo	TOO-lo
Stroke	estrok	es-TROK
Ulcer	ulser	OOL-ser
Ulcerative colitis	impeksion sa bituka	eem-pek-SYON sa bee-TOO-ka
UTI	impeksion sa pag-ihi	eem-pek-SYON sa pag-EE-hee
BODY PARTS		
Abdomen	tiyan	tee-YAN
Ankle	bukong-bukong	boo-KONG-boo-KONG
Appendix	apendiks	a-pen-DEEKS

Tagalog (Filipino)—Tagalog

Arm	braso	BRA-so
Artery	ugat / arterya	oo-GAT / ar-TE-ree-ya
Back	likod	lee-KOD
Bladder	pantug	pan-TOOG
Blood	dugo	doo-GO
Bone	buto	boo-TO
Brain	utak	OO-tak
Breast	suso	SOO-so
Calf	likod ng binti? (back of the leg)	lee-KOD ng been-TE?
Chest	dibdib	deeb-DEEB
Chin	baba	BA-ba
Ear	tenga	TE-nga
Elbow	siko	SEE-ko
Eye	mata	ma-TA
Face	mukha	mook-HA
Finger	daliri	da-LEE-ree
Foot	paa	pa-A
Hand	kamay	ka-MAY
Head	ulo	OO-lo
Heart	puso	POO-so
Gallbladder	apdo	ap-DO
Jaw	panga	pa-NGA
Joint	kasukasuan	ka-soo-ka-SOO-an
Kidney	bato	ba-TO
Knee	tuhod	TOO-hod
Leg	binti	been-TE

(cont.)

Liver	atay	a-TAY
Mouth	bibig	bee-BEEG
Muscle	kalamnan	ka-lam-NAN
Neck	leeg	lee-EG
Nerve	nerbyo	NER-bee-yo
Nose	ilong	ee-LONG
Ovary	obario	o-BAR-yoo
Pancreas	lapay	LA-pay
Penis	titi	TEE-tee
Prostate	prostate	pros-TA-te
Rectum	tumbong	toom-BONG
Rib	tadyang	tad-YANG
Shoulder	balikat	ba-LEE-kat
Skin	balat	ba-LAT
Spleen	esplin	es-PLEEN
Spine	buto sa likod	boo-TO sa lee-KOD
Stomach	sikmura	seek-MOO-ra
Teeth	ngipin	NGEE-peen
Testicle	bayag	ba-YAG
Throat	lalamunan	la-la-MOO-nan
Thyroid	tayroid	TAY-royd
Toe	daliri sa paa	da-LEE-ree sa pa-A
Tonsils	tonsil	TON-seel
Tongue	dila	DEE-la
Uterus	bahay-bata / matris	BA-hay-BA-ta /ma-TREES
Vagina	ari	A-ree
Vein	ugat	oo-GAT

| Wrist | galanggalangan | ga-lang-ga-LA-ngan |

NUMBERS

How many (times)?	ilang beses?	ee-LANG BE-ses?
0	sero	SE-ro
1	isa	ee-SA
2	dalawa	da-la-WA
3	tatlo	tat-LO
4	apat	A-pat
5	lima	lee-MA
6	anim	A-neem
7	pito	pee-TO
8	walo	wa-LO
9	siyam	see-YAM
10	sampu	sam-POO
11	labing isa	la-BEENG ee-SA
20	dalawampu	da-la-wam-POO
30	tatlompu	tat-lom-POO
40	apatnapu	A-pat-na-POO
50	limampu	lee-mam-POO
60	animnapu	A-neem-na-POO
70	pitumpu	pee-toom-POO
80	walumpu	wa-loom-POO
90	siyamnapu	see-yam-na-POO
100	isang daan	ee-SANG da-AN

Thai – ภาษาไทย

WORD/PHRASE	TRANSLATION	ENGLISH PRONUNCIATION
Thai	ภาษาไทย	pa-saa tay
INTRODUCTION & REGISTRATION		
Hello	สวัสดี ครับ/ค่ะ	sa-wat dee (krup - if speaker is male) / (ka - female)
I am doctor / nurse (add your name)	ฉันเป็นแพทย์ หมอ/พยาบาล ชื่อ (add your name)	chan b-pen maw / pa-ya-ban, CHU (add your name)
What is your name?	คุณชื่ออะไร?	koon CHU a-lay?
Who is your doctor?	ใครเป็นแพทย์ของคุณหมอของคุณ?	klay b-pen maw kong koon?
How old are you?	คุณอายุเท่าไหร่?	koon a-YOO TAU-lay?
Birthdate?	วันเดือนปีเกิด	wan du-an b-pee gert?
Telephone number?	เบอร์โทรศัพท์	ber to-ra-sap?
Address?	ที่อยู่	TEE-yoo?
Social security number?	เบอร์โซเชี่ยล	ber so-SH-YAL?
Insurance?	ประกันสุขภาพ	mee pra-gun sook-ga-PAP may?
BASICS		
Do you understand?	เข้าใจไหม	KAU-jay may?
Yes	ครับ(ค่ะ)	krup (M) / ka (F)
No	ไม่ ครับ(ค่ะ)	MAY krup (M) / MAY ka (F)
Please	กรุณา	ga-roo-naa
Thank you	ขอบคุณ	kawb koon krup (M) / ka (F)

(cont.)

Sorry	ขอโทษ	kaw-TOT
I don't understand	ไม่เข้าใจ	MAY KAU jay
Repeat	พูดอีกที	POOD eek tee
Speak slowly	พูดช้าๆ	POOD cha chaa
Answer "yes" or "no"	ตอบใช่หรือไม่ใช่	thawp "CHAY" lu "MAY CHAY"
Here	ตรงนี้	throng-NEE
This	อันนี้	an-NEE
It's alright (consoling)	ไม่เป็นไร	MAY b-pen lay
I'll be right back	เดี๋ยวกลับมา	dee-o glab maa
GENERAL		
What's wrong?	เป็นอะไร	b-pen a-lay
Pain	เจ็บ	jep
Do you have pain?	เจ็บไหม	jep may?
Does the pain radiate?	เจ็บไปถึงตรงไหน?	jep b-pay tung throng nay?
Where (show me)	ที่ไหน?	TEE nay?
Gone now	หายแล้ว	hay læw
Still present	ยังอยู่	yang yoo / yang mee
Sudden/gradual onset	เป็นทันที/ค่อยๆเป็น	b-pen tan-tee / KOY KOY b-pen
What bothers you the most?	มีอาการอะไรมากที่สุด	mee a-gan a-lay MAAK TEE soot
Why did you come today?	วันนี้มาทำอะไร	wan NEE maa tam a-lay?

QUALITY		
If '0' is no pain and 10 is maximum pain, what number do you have now?	ถ้าศูนย์ไม่เจ็บ,และสิบเจ็บมากที่สุด,คุณมีความเจ็บมากเท่าไหร่	TA SOON MAY jep, læw sip jep MAK TEE soot, koon mee kwam jep MAK TAU lay
Burning sensation	รู้สึกปวดแสบปวดร้อน	ROO suk b-poo-adt sæb b-poo-adt RON
Constant	ตลอดเวลา	tha-lawd wey-laa
Dull	ปวด	b-poo-adt
Intermittent pain	บางทีเจ็บ,บางทีไม่เจ็บ	bang tee jep, bang tee MAY jep
Pressure-like pain	เจ็บเหมือนโดนกด	jep mu-an don go-dt
Severe pain	เจ็บมากมาก	jep MAAK MAAK
Sharp/prickly pain	เจ็บแปล๊บแปล๊บ	jep PLÆB PLÆB
Throbbing	ปวดตุ๊บตุ๊บ	b-poo-adt thoop thoop
ASSOCIATED SYMPTOMS		
Onset during…(before/after)	เริ่มตอน…(ก่อน/หลัง)	LERM thawn… (gon / lung)
Worse (with…)	รู้สึกแย่ลง (ถ้า…)	LOO suk yæ long (TAA…)
Better (with…)	รู้สึกดีขึ้น (ถ้า…)	LOO suk dee KUN (TAA…)
Cough	ไอ	ay
Deep breath	หายใจลึกลึก	hay jay LUK LUK
Emotional upset	ไม่สบายใจ	MAY sa-bay jay
Eating	กินอาหาร	gkeen a-haan
Movement	ขยับ	ka-yup

(cont.)

Nothing	อยู่เฉยเฉย	yoo chu-y chu-y
Positioning	เปลี่ยนท่า	ple-an TAA
Rest	นอน	non
Walking	เดิน	durn
TIME COURSE		
For how long?	นานเท่าไหร่?	naan TAO lay?
Today	วันนี้	wan NEE
Yesterday	เมื่อวานนี้	MUA-wan NEE
How many...	กี่...	gee..
Months/weeks/days/hours/seconds	เดือน/อาทิตย์/วัน/ชั่วโมง/วินาที	duan/a-TIT/wan/chua-mong/WI-na-tee
Still present?	ยังรู้สึกอยู่ไหม?	yung LOO-SUK yoo may?
Gone now?	หายหรือยัง?	hay lu yung?
How long did it last? (see Numbers)	เป็นนานเท่าไหร่?	b-pen nan TAU lay?
Have you had this before?	เคยเป็นมาก่อนไหม?	kuy b-pen ma gon may?
How many times?	เป็นกี่ครั้ง?	b-pen gee KLUNG?
When was the last time?	ครั้งที่แล้วเป็นเมื่อไหร่?	KLUNG TEE laew b-pen MUA-lay?
New	ใหม่	may
Old	เก่า	gao
CONTEXT		
Did you...?	...ไหม?	...may?
fall	หกล้ม	hok-LOM?
trip	สะดุด	sa doodt?
faint	เป็นลม	b-pen lom?

twist	พลิก	plik
get hit	โดนทุบ ตี	don TOOP thee?
get burned	โดนไหม้	don MAY?
get assaulted	โดนทำร้าย	DON TAM-LAY?
get bitten	โดนกัด	don gadt?

PAST MEDICAL HISTORY

Take medication?	กินยาอะไรอยู่ไหม?	gin yaa alay yoo may?
(aspirin / antibiotics)	ยาแก้ปวด / ยาแก้อักเสบ	yaa GÆ b-poo-adt / yaa GÆ ak-seyb
Do you have (see Medical Problems)	มี...ไหม?	mee...MAY?
allergies	แพ้ยา	PÆ yaa
medical problems	โรคประจำตัว	LOK PRAJUM THOO-A
...problems of the (see Body Parts)	ปัญหาเกี่ยวกับ...	b-pan-haa gee-o gap...

SURGICAL HISTORY

Have you had surgery?	เคยผ่าตัดไหม?	KUY PAA-THUT MAY?
Surgery on...(see Body Parts)	ผ่าตัดที่...	paa-thut TEE...

SOCIAL HISTORY

Smoke?	สูบบุหรี่ไหม?	soob boo-lee may?
Drink? (Liquor/Beer)	กิน เหล้า/เบียร์ ไหม?	gin LAO / beea may?
Take drugs?	ใช้ยาเสพติดไหม?	CHAY yaa seyb-thit may?
Recent travel?	เพิ่งกลับจากเดินทางไหม?	PUNG glap jak durn tang may?
Are you sexually active?	ยังมีเซ็กซ์อยู่ไหม?	yung mee SEK yoo MAY?

(cont.)

Do you use condoms?	ใช้ถุงยางอนามัยไหม?	CHAY TOONG YANG AN-NA-MAY MAY?
Homosexual	เป็นรักร่วมเพศไหม	b-pen raak roo-aam peydt may?

SYSTEMS REVIEW

Do you have...	"มี...ไหม?	mee....may?

GENERAL

Fever	ไข้	KAY
Chills	ครั่นเนื้อครั่นตัว	KRAN nu-AA KRAN thoo-a
Weight loss	น้ำหนักลด	NAM-nak lodt
Fatigue	เหนื่อยไหม	NUY MAY?
Any sick contacts?	อยู่ใกล้ชิดกับคนไม่สบายไหม?	yoo GLAY chit gap kon MAY sa-bay may?

HEENT

Sore throat	คอเจ็บ	kaw jep
Runny nose	น้ำมูกไหล	NAM MOOG lay
Nosebleed	เลือดกำเดาไหล	lu-edt gam dao lay
Ear pain	เจ็บหู	jep hoo
EAR RINGING	หูแว่ว	HOO WÆ-W
Decreased hearing	หูได้ยินไม่ชัด	hoo DAI yin MAY SHUT

EYE

Eye pain	ตาเจ็บ	thaa jep
Blurry vision	ตาพร่ามัว	thaa PLA moo-a
Diplopia	เห็นภาพซ้อน	hen PAAB sawn
Foreign body sensation	รู้สึกมีอะไรในตา	ROO-SUK MEE A-LAY NAY THAA

Contact lenses	คอนแทคเลนส์	kon-tak len
CARDIAC		
Chest pain	เจ็บหน้าอก	jep NA-ok
Palpitations	หัวใจเต้น	hoo-A jay THEN
Orthopnea	หายใจไม่ออกตอนนอนหงาย	hay jay MAY auk thon non ngay
Dyspnea on exertion	หายใจไม่ออกตอนออกกำลังกาย	hay jay MAY auk thon auk gam-lung gay
Fainting (syncope)	เป็นลม	b-pen lom
Leg swelling	ขาบวม	KAA BOO-AM
How many pillows?	เวลานอน,ใช้หมอนกี่ใบ?	wey-laa non, chay mon gee bay?
PULMONARY		
Trouble breathing	ปัญหาเรื่องหายใจขัด	b-pun-haa lu-ANG hay jay kat
SOB	หายใจไม่ออก	hay jay MAY auk
Cough	ไอ	ay
Sputum	เสมหะ	seym-HA
Pain on inspiration	เจ็บตอนหายใจ	JEP THON HAY JAY
Hemoptysis	เลือดออกตอนไอ	lu-edt auk thon ay
GI		
Abdominal pain	ปวดท้อง	b-poo-adt TONG
Nausea	คลื่นไส้	kru-AN SAY
Vomiting	อาเจียน	a jee-en
Vomiting blood	อาเจียนเป็นเลือด	a jee-en b-pen lu-edt

(cont.)

Coffee ground emesis	อาเจียนเป็นสีน้ำตาลเหมือนกาแฟ	a jee-en b-pen see NAM-than mu-an ga-fæ
Anorexia	เป็นโรคกังวลเรื่องอ้วน	b-pen LOK gang-won lu-ANG oo-WAN
Diarrhea	ท้องเสีย	TONG see-A
Difficulty swallowing	กลืนลำบาก	glun lam-bak
BRBPR	มีเลือดในอุจจาระ	mee lu-edt nay ooj-ja-ra
Melena	อุจจาระสีดำ	ooj-ja-ra see dam
Pain after eating	ปวดท้องหลังอาหาร	b-poo-adt TONG lung a-haan
Worms	มีพยาธิ	MEE PA-YAAD
Constipation	ท้องผูก	TONG poogk
GU		
Painful urination	เจ็บเวลาฉี่	jep wey-laa chee
Urgent urination	ปวดปัสสาวะมากมาก	b-poo-adt b-plas-sa-wa MAAK MAAK
Frequent urination	ปัสสาวะบ่อย	b-plas-sa-wa boy
Bloody urination	มีเลือดในฉี่	MEE LU-EDT NAY CHEE
Discharge: vaginal/penile	ตกขาว	thok ka-O
PSYCH		
Anxiety	กังวล	gung-won
Depression	ซึมเศร้า	sum SAO
Suicidal thoughts	อยากฆ่าตัวตาย	yaak KAA thoo-a thay
Homicidal thoughts	อยากฆ่าคน...	yaak KAA kon un
Medication overdose	กินยาเกินขนาด	GKEEN YAA GURN KA-NAAD
Hear voices	ชูหว่าได้ยินคนพูด	hoo wæw DAY yin kon POOD

NEURO		
Headache	ปวดหัว	b-poo-adt hoo-A
Worst headache of life	ปวดหัวมากที่สุดในชีวิต	b-poo-adt hoo-A MAAK TEE soot nay shee-WIT
Weakness	ไม่มีแรง	MAY mee læng
Dizzy	เวียนหัว	wee-an hoo-A
What is your name?	คุณชื่ออะไร?	koon CHU a-lay?
Where are we?	เราอยู่ที่ไหน?	lao yoo TEE nay?
What is the year/month/date?	ปีนี้ปีอะไร?/เดือนนี้เดือนอะไร?/วันนี้วันอะไร?	b-pee NEE b-pee a-lay? / duan NEE duan a-lay? / wan NEE wan a-lay?
Bowel dysfunction	ปัญหาเรื่องอุจจาระ	b-pun-haa lu-ANG ooj-ja-ra
Bladder dysfunction	ปัญหาเรื่องปัสสาวะ	b-pun-haa lu-ANG b-plas-sa-wa
Photophobia	เจ็บตาตอนเห็นแสงสว่าง	jep thaa thon hen sæng sa-wang
Tingling/numbness	เป็นเหน็บ/ชา	b-pen nep / chaa
Decreased strength in... (See Body Part List)	(อวัยวะ) อ่อนแรง	(body part) awn læng
Seizure	ชัก	shuk
Difficulty walking	ปัญหาเรื่องเดิน	bun-haa ru-ANG durn
Difficulty speaking	ปัญหาเวลาพูด	bun-haa wey-laa POOD
Spinning (vertigo)	หัวหมุน	hoo-A moon
Confusion	หลง	long
MISC		
Lump	เนื้องอก	nu-AA NGOK

(cont.)

Itching	คัน	kun
Bruising	รอยช้ำ	loy CHUM
Rash	เป็นผื่น	b-pen pun
Swelling	บวม	boo-am
Jaundice	ตัวเหลือง	thoo-a lu-ANG

GYNECOLOGIC

Vaginal bleeding	เลือดออกทางช่องคลอด	lu-edt auk tang CHONG KLOD
Heavy	มาก	MAAK
Irregular	ไม่ปกติ	MAY bok-ka-thi
Absent	ไม่มีเมนส์	MAY mee men
Vaginal discharge	ตกขาว	thok ka-O
Pelvic pain	เจ็บท้องน้อย	jep TONG NOY
Rape	ข่มขืน	kom kurn
Pain with intercourse	เจ็บเวลามีเซ็กซ์	jep wey-laa mee SEK
Contraceptive	คุมกำเนิด	koom gam nerdt

OBSTETRIC

Are you pregnant?	กำลังท้องไหม?	gum lung TONG may?
LMP how many days ago?	เมนส์ครั้งสุดท้ายเมื่อไหร่?	mee men KLANG soot-TAY MU-A lay?
Times pregnant?	ท้องกี่ครั้ง?	TONG gee KLANG?
Times delivered?	คลอดกี่ครั้ง?	KLOD gee KLANG?
Miscarriage	แท้ง	TÆNG
Abortion	ทำแท้ง	tam TÆNG
Fluid leakage	ถุงน้ำคร่ำแตก	toong NAM krum thæk

Contraction	มดลูกบีบตัว	MOT LOOGK beep tua
Fetal movement	เด็กขยับตัว	dek ka-yup thoo-a
TRAUMA		
How many hours ago did you eat last?	กินข้าวกี่ชั่วโมงก่อนมานี่?	gin KAO gee chua-mong gon maa NEE?
Lost consciousness?	สลบหรือไม่?	sa-lop lu may?
Tetanus within 5 years?	ภายในห้าปีก่อน,เคยฉีดยาบาดทะยักไหม?	pay nay HAA b-pee gon, kuy cheedt yaa badt-ta-yuk may?
PEDIATRIC		
How old?	อายุเท่าไหร่?	a-YOO tao lay?
Vaccines up to date?	ฉีดวัคซีนครบไหม?	cheedt VAK-seen KLOP may?
Urinating normally	ฉี่ปกติ	chee bok-ka-thi
Taking liquids	ดื่มน้ำ	dum NAM
Increased crying	ร้องให้มากขึ้น	LONG-HAY MAAK KUN
Ingestion	กินของแปลกปลอม	gkeen kong b-plæk b-plom
Foreign body	ของแปลกปลอมใส่ตัว	gkeen kong b-plæk b-plom say thoo-a
Premature	คลอดก่อนกำหนด	KLOD gon gum nodt
Birth complications	ปัญหาตอนคลอด	b-pun-haa thon KLOD
PHYSICAL EXAM/INSTRUCTION		
Sit down (please)	โปรดนั่ง	b-plod NUNG
Lie down	โปรดนอนลง	b-plod nawn long
Come here	มานี่	maa NEE

(cont.)

Relax	รีแลกซ์	re-lak
Don't move	ไปรดอย่าขยับ	b-plod yaa ka-yap
Open your mouth	อ้าปาก	AA b-pak
Say "ahh"	ทำเสียง"อา"	tam see-eng "ahh"
Swallow	กลืน	glun
Breath deeply	หายใจลึกลึก	hay jay luk-luk
Hold your breath	กลั้นหายใจ	GLUN hay jay
Cough	ไอ	ay
Push	ผลัก	pluk
Pull	ดึง	dung
Follow my finger with your eyes	มองตามนิ้ว	mong tham ni-OO
Close your eyes	ปิดตา	b-pit thaa
Smile	ยิ้ม	YIM
Can you feel this?	รู้สึกไหม?	LOO-suk may?
Copy this (movement)	ทำตามฉัน	tam thaam chan
I am going to put a finger in your rectum	ฉันจะใช้นิ้วตรวจช่องทวาร	chan ja chay ni-OO throo-adt CHONG ta-wan
I am going to examine your vagina	ฉันจะตรวจช่องคลอด	chan ja throo-adt CHONG KLOD
REASSESSMENT		
Do you feel better?	รู้สึกดีขึ้นไหม?	LOO-suk dee KUN may?
Do you feel worse?	รู้สึกแย่ลงไหม?	LOO-suk YÆ long may?

PATIENT WORDS		
I hurt	เจ็บ	jep
Help!	ช่วยด้วย	CHOO-AY doo-AY!
Bathroom	ห้องน้ำ	hong NAM
Food	อาหาร	aa-haan
Water	น้ำ	NAM
PROCEDURES & CONSENT		
You need...	คุณต้องการ...	koon THONG gaan...
Injection	ฉีดยา	cheedt yaa
Stiches	เย็บแผล	YEP pæ
Cast	เฝือก	fu-ak
Crutches	ไม้พยุงตัว	MAY pa-yoong thoo-a
Perform surgery on... (See Body Parts)	ผ่าตัด...	paa-that...
The risks are...	ความเสี่ยงคือ	kwam see-ang ku
Bleeding	เลือดไหล	lu-edt lay
Infection	อักเสบ	ak-seyb
Scar	แผลเป็น	plæ b-pen
Repeat procedure	ทำขั้นตอนซ้ำอีก	tam KAN-thon SUM eeg
Iodine	ไอโอดีน	AY-o-deen
Damage to (see Body Parts)	(อวัยวะ)บาดเจ็บ	(body part) baad jep
Sign here	เซ็นชื่อตรงนี้	sen CHU throng NEE

(cont.)

TESTS		
X-ray	เอ็กซเรย์	eks-rey
C.A.T. Scan	แคทสแกน	KAT skæn
Ultrasound	อุลตราซาวน์	ool-thra-sau
Catheterization/bladder catheter	สวนปัสสาวะ	soo-an b-plas-sa-wa
Colonoscopy	ส่องกล้องลำไส้ใหญ่	song GLONG lum SAY
Endoscopy	ส่องกล้องทางปาก	song GLONG tang b-paak
END OF LIFE		
Do you want us to...	คุณต้องการให้พวกเราทำ...	koon thong gan HAY pu-AK lao tum...
Perform CPR	ซีพีอาร์	see pee aa
Defibrillate	ช็อตหัวใจ	SHODT hoo-A jay
Intubate	ใส่ท่อช่วยหายใจ	say TAW choo-AY hay-jay
He/she is dead	เขาเสียแล้ว	kao see-A læw
We did all we could	เราทำเต็มที่แล้ว	lao tam them-TEE læw
DISCHARGE		
You have...(See Medical Prob List)	คุณมี / เป็น...	koon mee / b-pen...
He/she is going to stay in the hospital	เขาต้องการพักในโรงพยาบาล	kao THONG gan PAK nay long-pa-ya baan
Take "X" pills "Y" times a day (for "Z" days)	กิน_เม็ด ครั้งต่อวัน(สำหรับ_วัน)	gkeen "X" MET "Y" KRANG thaw wan (sam lup "Z" wan)
Pills	เม็ด	MET
Antibiotics	ยาแก้อักเสบ	yaa GÆ ak-seyb
Before/after meals	ก่อน/หลัง อาหาร	gon/lung a-haan

Return to the ER if…	กลับมาที่แผนกฉุกเฉินถ้า…	glab maa TEE long-pa-ya-ban TAA…
Follow up at "X" on "Y"	กลับมาตรวจ (ที่) (วัน)	glab maa throo-adt TEE "X", "Y"
You're welcome	ไม่เป็นไร	MAY b-pen lay
Goodbye	สวัสดี ครับ/ค่ะ	sa-wat-dee krup/ka
MEDICAL PROBS		
AIDS/HIV	เอดส์	eyd
Anemia	โลหิตจาง	LO-heet jaang
Arrhythmia	หัวใจเต้นไม่ปกติ	hoo-A jay THEN MAY bok-ka-thi
Arthritis	ปวดตามข้อ	b-poo-adt tham KAW
Asthma	หอบ	hob
Bronchitis	หลอดลมอักเสบ	lodt lom ak-seyb
Cancer	มะเร็ง	ma-leng
Cirrhosis	โรคตับ/ตับแข็ง	LOK thup / thup kæng
Cholesterol	คอเลสเตอรอล	ko-les-ther-ral
Cold	หวัด	wadt
Constipation	ท้องผูก	TONG poogk
Cyst	ซีส	sis
Diabetes	เบาหวาน	bau-waan
Dialysis	ฟอกไต	FOG thay
Diverticulitis	ถุงตันที่ลำไส้ใหญ่อักเสบ	toong tan tee lum SAY yay ak-seyb
Emphysema	ถุงลมปอดโป่งพอง	toong lom bawdt pong pong

(cont.)

Fibroids	เนื้องอกในมดลูก	nu-AA NGOK nay MOT LOOGK
Fracture	กระดูกร้าว	gra-dook LAO
Flu	ไข้หวัด	KAY-wadt
Gallstones	นิ่วในถุงน้ำดี	ni-OO nay toong NAM dee
Gastritis/GERD	กระเพาะอาหารอักเสบ	gra-PAU a-haan ak-seyb
Hepatitis	ตับอักเสบ	thup ak-seyb
Heart attack	หัวใจวาย	hoo-A jay way
Heart disease	โรคหัวใจ	LOK hoo-A jay
Heart failure	หัวใจล้มเหลว	hoo-A jay LOM ley-oo
Hypertension	ความดันสูง	kwam dun soong
Indigestion	อาหารไม่ย่อย	a-haan MAY YOY
Kidney stone	นิ่วในไต	ni-OO nay thay
Lupus	โรคภูมิแพ้ตัวเอง	LOK poom pæ thoo-a eng
Migraine	ไมเกรน	may-greyn
Murmur	เสียงเต้นหัวใจไม่ปกติ	see-eng THEN hoo-A jay MAY b-pok-ka-thi
Pacemaker	เครื่องช่วยหัวใจทำงาน	klu-UNG shoo-AY hoo-A jay tam ngan
Pneumonia	นิวโมเนีย	niw-mon-ni-aa
Epilepsy	โรคลมชัก	LOK lom shuk
STD	โรคติดต่อทางเพศสัมพันธ์	LOK thit thaw tang peyd sum-pun
Stroke	การอุดตันของเส้นเลือดที่เลี้ยงสมอง	gaan oot-thun kong SEN lu-edt TEE lee-eng sa-mong
Ulcer	แผลในกระเพาะ	plæ nay gra-PAU

Ulcerative colitis	ลำไส้ใหญ่อักเสบ	lum SAY yay ak-seyb
UTI	ทางเดินปัสสาวะอักเสบ	tang doen b-plas-sa-wa ak-seyb

BODY PARTS

Abdomen	ท้อง	TONG
Ankle	ข้อเท้า	KAW ta-o
Appendix	ไส้ติ่ง	SAY thing
Arm	แขน	kæn
Artery	เส้นเลือดแดง	SEN lu-edt dæng
Back	หลัง	lung
Bladder	กระเพาะปัสสาวะ	b-plas-sa-wa
Blood	เลือด	lu-edt
Bone	กระดูก	gra-dook
Brain	สมอง	sa-mong
Breast	เต้านม	tha-o nom
Calf	น่อง	NONG
Chest	หน้าอก	NAA-ok
Chin	คาง	kang
Ear	หู	hoo
Elbow	ข้อศอก	KAW SOK
Eye	ตา	thaa
Face	หน้า	NAA
Finger	นิ้ว	ni-OO

(cont.)

Foot	เท้า	TA-O
Hand	มือ	mu
Head	หัว	hoo-A
Heart	หัวใจ	hoo-A jay
Gallbladder	ถุงน้ำดี	toong NAM dee
Jaw	กราม	graam
Joint	ข้อต่อ	KAW thaw
Kidney	ไต	thay
Knee	เข่า	kow
Leg	ขา	kaa
Liver	ตับ	thup
Mouth	ปาก	b-paak
Muscle	กล้ามเนื้อ	GLAAM nu-AA
Neck	คอ	kaw
Nerve	เส้นประสาท	SEN pra-saat
Nose	จมูก	ja-moogk
Ovary	รังไข่	lung kay
Pancreas	ตับอ่อน	thup on
Penis	องคชาต	ong-ka-chaat
Prostate	ต่อมลูกหมาก	thom loogk maa-gk
Rectum	ช่องทวาร	CHONG ta-wan
Rib	ซี่โครง	see krong
Shoulder	ไหล่	lay

Skin	ผิวหนัง	pi-OO-nung
Spleen	ม้าม	MAAM
Spine	กระดูกสันหลัง	gra-dook sun lung
Stomach	กระเพาะ	gra-PAU
Teeth	ฟัน	fun
Testicle	ลูกหมาก	LOOGK maa-gk
Throat	คอ	kaw
Thyroid	ไทรอยด์	thay-roy
Toe	นิ้วเท้า	ni-OO TAU
Tonsils	ทอนซิล	ton sin
Tongue	ลิ้น	LIN
Uterus	มดลูก	modt LOOGK
Vagina	ช่องคลอด	CHONG KLOD
Vein	เส้นเลือดดำ	SEN lu-edt dam
Wrist	ข้อมือ	KAW mu

(cont.)

NUMBERS

How many (times)?	กี่ครั้ง	gee KLANG?
0	ศูนย์	soon
1	หนึ่ง	nung
2	สอง	song
3	สาม	sam
4	สี่	see
5	ห้า	HAA
6	หก	hok
7	เจ็ด	jet
8	แปด	bædt
9	เก้า	GAU
10	สิบ	sip
11	สิบเอ็ด	sip et
20	ยี่สิบ	YEE sip
30	สามสิบ	sam sip
40	สี่สิบ	see sip
50	ห้าสิบ	HAA sip
60	หกสิบ	hok sip
70	เจ็ดสิบ	jet sip
80	แปดสิบ	bædt sip
90	เก้าสิบ	GAU SIP
100	หนึ่งร้อย	NUNG LOY

Ukrainian — Українська мова

WORD/PHRASE	TRANSLATION	ENGLISH PRONUNCIATION
Ukrainian	Українська мова	oo-kra-YEEN-ska MO-va
INTRODUCTION & REGISTRATION		
Hello	Добрий день	DOB-ree den
I am a doctor / nurse	Я лікар / медсестра *(fem)* медбрат *(masc)*	ya LEE-kar (doctor) / med-ses-TRA *(fem)* med-BRAT *(masc)*
What is your name?	Як вас звати?	yak vas z-VA-ti?
Who is your doctor?	Хто Ваш лікар?	kh-TO vash LEE-kar?
How old are you?	Скільки Вам років?	SKEEL-ki vam RO-keew?
Birthdate?	Число народження?	chis-LO na-RO-jen-nya?
Telephone number?	Нумер телефону?	NOO-mer te-LE-fo-noo?
Address?	Адреса?	ad-RE-sa?
Social security number?	Нумер соціального забезпечення?	NOO-mer so-tsee-al-no-ho za-bez-PE-chen-nya?
Insurance?	Страхування?	stra-kho-VAN-nya?
BASICS		
Do you understand?	Чи ви розумієте?	chi vi ro-zoo-MEE-ye-te?
Yes	Так	tak
No	Ні	nee
Please	Прошу	PRO-shoo

(cont.)

Thank you	Дякую	D-YA-koo-yoo
Sorry	Перепрошую	pe-re-PRO-shoo-yoo
I don't understand	Я не розумію	ya ne ro-zoo-MEE-yoo
Repeat	Прошу повторити	PRO-shoo pov-to-RI-ti
Speak slowly	Говоріть повільно	ho-vo-REET po-VEEL-no
Answer "yes" or "no"	Відповідайте «так» або «ні»	veed-po-vee-DAY-te "tak" a-bo "nee"
Here	Тут	toot
This	Це	tse
It's alright (consoling)	Все в порядку	v-se v po-ryad-koo
I'll be right back	Я вже вернуся	ya v-zhe ver-NOO-s-ya
GENERAL		
What's wrong?	Що трапилось?	sh-cho TRA-pi-los?
Pain	Біль	beel
Do you have pain?	Чи вам болить?	chi vam bo-LIT
Does the pain radiate?	Чи біль випромінює кудись?	chi beel vi-pro-meen-YOO-ye koo-DIS?
Where (show me)	Де? Покажіть мені	DE? po-ka-ZHEET me-NEE
Gone now	Вже нема	v-zhe ne-MA
Still present	Ще є	sh-CHE ye
Sudden/gradual onset	Раптом / поступово	RAP-tom / po-stoo-PO-vo
What bothers you the most?	Що вам заважає найбільше?	sh-cho vam za-va-ZHA-ye nay-BEEL-she?
Why did you come today?	Чому ви сьогодні прийшли?	cho-MOO vi s-yo-HOD-nee preesh-LI?

QUALITY		
If '0' is no pain and 10 is maximum pain, what number do you have now?	Якщо нуль означає ніякий біль, та десять є найстрашний біль, котрий нумер ви маєте тепер?	yak-sh-CHO NOOL oz-na-CHA-ye nee-YA-kee beel, ta DES-yat ye nay-STRASH-nee beel, ko-TREE NOO-mer vi MA-ye-te-PER?
Burning	Пекучий	pe-KOO-chee
Constant	Постійний	po-STEE-nee
Dull	Тупий	too-PEE
Intermittent	Переривчастий	pe-re-riv-CHAS-tee
Pressure	Тисковий	tis-KO-vee
Severe	Страшний	strash-NEE
Sharp/prickly pains	Гострий	HOS-tree
Throbbing	Біль, який пульсує	beel, ya-KEE pool-SOO-ye
ASSOCIATED SYMPTOMS		
Onset during... (before/after)	Почалось протягом...(перед/після)	po-CHA-los pro-t-ya-HOM...(PE-red/PEES-l-ya)
Worse (with...)	Гірше коли...	HEER-she ko-LI...
Better (with...)	Краще коли...	KRA-sh-che ko-LI...
Cough	Кашляєте?	KASH-l-ya-ye-te?
Deep breath	Придихаєте глибоко?	pri-di-KHA-ye-te h-li-BO-ko?
Emotional upset	Розстроєні?	roz-STRO-ye-nee?
Food	Їсте?	YEES-te?
Movement	Рухаєтеся?	ROO-kha-ye-te-s-ya?

(cont.)

Nothing	Нічого не робите?	nee-CHO-ho ne RO-bi-te?
Positioning	Ви в будь-якому положенні?	vi v bood-ya-KO-moo po-LO-zhen-nee?
Rest	Відпочиваєте?	veed-po-chi-VA-ye-te?
Walking	Ходите?	KHO-di-te?

TIME COURSE

For how long?	Скільки часу?	SKEEL-ki cha-SOO?
Today	Сьогодні	s-yo-HOD-nee
Yesterday	Учора	oo-CHO-ra
How many...	Скільки...	SKEEL-ki
Months/weeks/days/hours/seconds	Місяців/тижнів/годин/секунд	MEES-yat-tseew *(months)* / TIZH-d-neew *(weeks)*/ ho-DIN *(hours)*/ se-KOON-D *(seconds)*
Still present?	Ще маєте?	sh-CHE MA-ye-te?
Gone now?	Тепер нема?	te-PER ne-MA?
How long did it last? (See Numbers List)	Скільки часу тривало це?	SKEEL-ki cha-SOO tri-VA-lo tse?
Have you had this before?	Вам колись так стало раніше?	vam ko-LIS tak STA-lo ra-NEE-she?
How many times?	Скільки разів?	SKEEL-ki ra-ZEEW?
When was the last time?	Коли був останній раз?	ko-LI boov o-STAN-nee raz?
New	Нове	no-VE
Old	Старе	sta-PE

CONTEXT

Did you...?	Чи ви...	chi vi...

fall	Впали?	v-PA-li?
trip	Спіткнулись?	speet-k-NOO-lis?
faint	Зомліли?	zom-LEE-li?
twist	Скручувались?	s-kroo-choo-VA-lis?
get hit	Вдарились?	v-DA-ri-lis?
get burned	Спалились?	spa-LI-lis?
get assaulted	Були пошкоджені насильством?	BOO-li posh-KO-je-nee na-SIL-st-vom?
get bitten (human/dog/cat/insect)	Були покусані?	BOO-li po-KOO-sa-nee?
PAST MEDICAL HISTORY		
Take medication?	Приймаєте лікарство?	priy-MA-ye-te lee-KARST-vo?
(aspirin/antibiotics)	Аспирина/антибіотики	as-pi-RI-na/ an-ti-bee-O-ti-ki
Do you have (See also Medical Problem List)…	Чи ви маєте…	chi vi MA-ye-te…
allergies	Алергії?	a-LER-hee-yee?
medical problems	Медичні проблеми?	me-DICH-nee prob-LE-mi
Do you have problems of the…(see Body Parts List)	Чи ви маєте проблеми з…	chi vi MA-ye-te prob-LE-mi z…
SURGICAL HISTORY		
Have you had surgery?	Зробили вам операцію?	z-ro-BI-li vam o-pe-RA-tsee-yoo?
Surgery on/"to remove"…(see Body Parts List)	Операція на…	o-pe-RA-tsee-ya na…

(cont.)

SOCIAL HISTORY		
Smoke?	Курите?	KOO-ri-te?
Drink?	П'єте алкоголь?	p-YE-te al-ko-HOL?
Take drugs?	Приймаєте наркотики?	priy-MA-ye-te nar-KO-ti-ki?
Recent travel?	Мандрували недавно?	man-droo-VA-li ne-DAV-no?
Are you sexually active?	Займаєтеся сексом з кимось?	zay-MA-ye-te-s-ya SEK-som z KIM-os?
Do you use condoms?	Уживаєте презервативи / кондоми?	oo-zhi-VA-ye-te pre-ser-va-TI-vi / kon-DO-mi?
Homosexual	Гомосексуаліст?	ho-mo-sek-soo-a-LEEST?
SYSTEMS REVIEW		
Do you have...	Чи у вас..	chi oo vas...
GENERAL		
Fever	Гарячка?	Har-YACH-ka?
Chills	Дрожі?	DRO-zhee?
Weight loss	Втрачання ваги?	v-tra-CHAN-nya va-HI?
Fatigue	Утомлення?	oo-TOM-len-nya?
Sick contact	Контакт з захворенними?	kon-TAKT Z za-KH-VO-re-ni-mi
HEENT		
Sore throat	Хворе горло	kh-VO-re HOR-lo
Runny nose	насмарк	NAS-mark
Nosebleed	Кров носом іде	krov NO-som ee-DE
Ear pain	Біль вуха	beel VOO-kha
Ear ringing	Дзвоніння у вухах	d-z-vo-NEEN-nya oo VOO-khakh

Decreased hearing	Пошкоджений слух	posh-KO-je-nee s-LOOKH
EYE		
Eye pain	Біль в очах	beel v o-CHAKH
Blurry vision	Нечіткий зір	ne-CHEET-kee zeer
Diplopia	Подвійний зір	po-D-VEE-niy zeer
Foreign body sensation	Відчуття чогось чужорідного в очах	veed-CHOOT-tya cho-HOS cho-zho-REED-no-ho v o-CHAKH
Contact lenses	Контактні лінзи	kon-TAK-T-nee LEEN-zi
CARDIAC		
Chest pain	Біль в грудях	beel v H-ROOD-yakh
Palpitations	Сильне серцебиття	SIL-ne ser-tse-BIT-tya
Orthopnea	Задихані, коли ви лежите?	za-DI-kha-nee, ko-LI vi le-ZHI-te?
Dyspnea on exertion	Задишка при фізичному напруженні	za-DISH-ka pri fee-ZICH-no-moo na-PROO-zhen-nee
Fainting (syncope)	Зомління	zom-LEEN-nya
Leg swelling	Спухлені ноги	s-POOKH-le-nee NO-hi
How many pillows?	Скільки подушок уживаєте, щоб краще дихати коли спите?	SKEEL-ki PO-doo-shok oo-zhi-VA-ye-te, sh-CHOB KRASH-che DI-kha-ti ko-LI spi-TE?
PULMONARY		
Trouble breathing	Тяжко дихати	T-YAZH-ko DI-kha-ti

(cont.)

SOB	Важкість дихання	VAZH-keest DI-khan-nya
Cough	Кашель	KA-shel
Sputum	Плювок	pl-yoo-VOK
Pain on inspiration	Біль, коли придихаєтеся?	beel, ko-LI pri-di-KHA-ye-te-s-ya?
Hemoptysis	Кровоточивий кашель	kro-vo-to-CHI-vee KA-shel
GI		
Abdominal pain	Біль в животі	Beel v zhi-vo-TEE
Nausea	Нудота	noo-do-TA
Vomiting	Блювання	b-l-yoo-VAN-nya
Vomiting blood	Блювання крови	b-l-yoo-VAN-nya KRO-vi
Coffee ground emesis	Блювання крови, що схоже на кавову гущу	b-l-yoo-VAN-nya KRO-vi, sh-cho s-kho-zhe na ka-VO-voo HOOSH-choo
Anorexia	Відситність апетиту	Veed-SOOT-neest a-pe-TI-too
Diarrhea	Пронос / Діярея	pro-NOS / dee-ya-RE-ya
Difficulty swallowing	Важкість ковтання	VAZH-keest kov-TAN-nya
BRBPR	Червона кров із заднього проходу	cher-VO-na krov eez ZAD-n-yo-ho PRO-kho-doo
Melena	Кал у вигляді липкої маси чорного кольору	kal oo VI-H-l-ya-dee lip-KO-yee MA-si CHOR-no-ho KO-lo-roo
Pain after eating	Біль після їжи	beel PEES-l-ya YEE-zhi
Worms	Глисти / Черв'яки	hlis-TY / cher-v-YA-ki

Constipation	Запор	ZA-por
GU		
Painful urination	Болюче / Пекуче сечовипускання	bo-LYOO-che / pe-KOO-che se-cho-vi-poos-KAN-nya
Urgent urination	Негайне сечовипускання	ne-HAY-ne se-cho-vi-poos-KAN-nya
Frequent urination	Часте сечовипускання	CHAS-te se-cho-vi-poos-KAN-nya
Bloody urination	Криваве сечовипускання	kri-VA-ve se-cho-vi-poos-KAN-nya
Discharge: vaginal/penile	Виділення: з вагіни (з піхви)/ з пеніса (зі статевого члена)	vi-DEE-len-nya: z VA-hee-ni (z PEEKH-vi) (vaginal) / z PE-nee-sa (zee sta-TE-vo-ho CHLE-na)(penile)
PSYCH		
Anxiety	Тривога	tri-VO-ha
Depression	Депресія	de-PRE-see-ya
Suicidal thoughts	Самогубні думки	sa-mo-HOOB-nee DOOM-ki
Homicidal thoughts	Убивчі думки	oo-BIV-chee DOOM-ki
Medication overdose	Надмірна доза	nad-MEER-na DO-za
Hear voices	Слухові галюцинації	sloo-KHO-vee ha-l-yoo-tsi-NA-tsee-yee
NEURO		
Headache	Біль голови	beel ho-lo-VI
Worst headache of life	Найгірший біль голови в житті	nay-HEER-shee beel ho-lo-VI v zhit-TEE
Weakness	слабкість	SLAB-keest

(cont.)

Dizzy	Запаморочення	za-pa-mo-RO-chen-nya
What is your name?	Як вас звати?	yak vas z-VA-ti?
Where are we?	Де ми?	DE mi?
What is the year/month/date?	Котрий тепер: рік/ місяць/ день?	Ko-TRIY te-PER: reek (year)/ MEES-yats' (month)/ den (year)?
Bowel dysfunction	Проблеми котролювати випороження	prob-LE-mi kon-tro-l-yoo-VA-ti vi-po-RO-zhen-nya
Bladder dysfunction	Проблеми котролювати сечовипускання	prob-LE-mi kon-tro-l-yoo-VA-ti se-cho-vi-poos-KAN-nya
Photophobia	Світобоязнь (підвищена чутливість ока до світла)	s-VEE-to-bo-YAZ-n (peed-VISH-chen-nya choot-LI-veest O-ka do s-VEET-la)
Tingling/ numbness	Поколювання / нечутливість	po-ko-l-yoo-VAN-nya / ne-choot-LI-veest
Decreased strength in... (See Body Parts List)	Зменшена сила в...	z-MEN-she-na SI-la v...
Seizure	Апоплексичний удар	a-po-plek-SICH-nee OO-dar
Difficulty walking	Важко ходити	VAZH-ko kho-DI-ti
Difficulty speaking	Важко говорити	VAZH-ko ho-vo-RI-ti
Spinning (vertigo)	Запаморочення	za-pa-mo-RO-chen-nya
Confusion	Плутанина	ploo-ta-NI-na
MISC		
Lump	Ґуля	GOOL-ya
Itching	Свербіння	s-ver-BEEN-nya

Bruising	Синяки	sin-ya-KI
Rash	Висип	VI-sip
Swelling	Опухлість	o-POOKH-leest
Jaundice (yellow skin)	Жовтяниця	zhov-t-YA-ni-ts-ya

GYNECOLOGIC

Vaginal bleeding	Кровотеча з вагіни (з піхви)	kro-vo-TE-cha z VA-hee-ni (z PEEKH-vi)
Heavy	Сильна	SIL-na
Irregular	Нерівна	ne-REEV-na
Absent	Відсутність менструації	veed-SOOT-neest men-stroo-A-tsee-yee
Vaginal discharge	Виділення з вагіни (з піхви)	vi-DEE-len-nya z VA-hee-ni (z PEEKH-vi)
Pelvic pain	Тазовий біль	taz-O-vee beel
Rape	Згвалтування	z-g-val-too-VAN-nya
Pain with intercourse	Біль під час статевого акту	beel peed chas sta-TE-vo-ho AK-too
Contraceptive	Протизаплідний засіб	pro-ti-za-PLEED-niy ZA-seeb

OBSTETRIC

Are you pregnant?	Чи ви вагітні?	chi vi va-HEET-nee?
LMP how many days ago?	Скільки днів назад була остання менструація?	SKEEL-ki d-neew na-ZAD BOO-la o-STAN-nya men-stroo-A-tsee-ya?
Times pregnant?	Скільки разів були вагітні?	SKEEL-ki ra-ZEEW BOO-li va-HEET-nee?
Times delivered?	Скільки народжень?	SKEEL-ki na-RO-jen?
Miscarriage	Викидень	vi-KI-den

(cont.)

Abortion	Аборт	a-BORT
Fluid leakage	Витік рідини	VI-teek ree-di-NI
Contraction	Перейми / Скорочення	pe-REY-mi / sko-RO-chen-nya
Fetal movement	Рух плоду / немовлі	rookh PLO-doo / ne-mov-LEE
TRAUMA		
How many hours ago did you eat last?	Скільки годин назад ви їли?	SKEEL-ki ho-DIN ha-ZAD vi YEE-li?
Lost consciousness?	Утратили свідомість?	oo-TRA-ti-li s-vee-DO-meest?
Tetanus within 5 years?	Щеплення проти тетануса за останні п'ять(5) років?	sh-CHEP-len-nya PRO-ti TE-ta-noo-sa za os-TAN-nee p-YAT RO-keew?
PEDIATRIC		
How old?	Скільки років (years)/ місяців (months)/ днів (days)?	SKEEL'-ki RO-keev (years) / MEES-ya-tseev (months)/ DNEEV (days)?
Vaccines up to date?	Щеплення нинішні?	SHCHEP-len-nya NI-neesh-nee?
Urinating normally	Мочиться добре?	MO-chit-sya DO-bre?
Taking liquids	Приймає рідини добре?	preey-MA-ye ree-DI-ni DO-bre?
Increased crying	Плакає більше?	PLA-ka-ye BEEL'-she?
Ingestion	Ковтання чогось чужорідного?	KOV-tan-nya
Foreign body	Чужорідний предмет	chu-zho-REED-niy pred-MET
Premature	Передчасне народження	ne-do-NO-she-niy

Birth complications	Ускладнення родів	oos-KLAD-nen-nya RO-div

PHYSICAL EXAM/INSTRUCTION

Sit down (please)	Прошу сісти	PRO-shoo SEES-ti
Lie down	Лягте	LYAH-TE
Come here	Прийдіть сюди	pree-DEET s-yoo-DI
Relax	Постарайтеся розслабитися	po-sta-RAY-te-s-ya roz-sla-BI-ti-s-ya
Don't move	Не рухайтеся	ne ROO-khay-tes-ya
Open your mouth	Відкрийте рот	veed-KREE-te rot
Say "ahh"	Скажіть «Ааа»	ska-ZHEET "Aaa"
Swallow	Ковтайте	kov-TAY-te
Breath deeply	Придихніть глибоко	pri-dikh-NEET' h-li-BO-ko
Hold your breath	Затримайте подих	za-TRI-may-te PO-dikh
Cough	Кашляйте	KASH-l-yay-te
Push	Пхайте	p-KHAY-te
Pull	Потягніть	po-t-ya-h-NEET
Follow my finger	Слідіть очима за моїм пальцем	slee-DEET o-CHI-ma za mo-YEEM PAL-tsem
Close your eyes	Закрийте очі	za-KRIY-te O-chee
Smile	Усміхайтесь	oo-smi-KHAY-tes
Can you feel this?	Відчуваєте це?	veed-choo-VA-ye-te tse?
Copy this (movement)	Робіть так.	ro-BEET tak
I am going to put a finger in your rectum	Я мушу покласти пальця в пряму кишку	ya MOO-shoo po-KLAS-ti PAL-ts-ya v p-r-YA-moo KISH-koo

(cont.)

I am going to examine your vagina	Я збадаю вагіну	ya z-BA-da-yoo VA-hee-noo
REASSESSMENT		
Do you feel better?	Краще себе почуваєте?	KRASH-che se-BE po-choo-VA-ye-te?
Do you feel worse?	Гірше себе почуваєте?	HEER-she se-BE po-choo-VA-ye-te?
PATIENT WORDS		
I hurt	Мені болить	me-NEE bo-LIT
Help!	Допоможіть!	do-po-mo-ZHEET!
Bathroom	Туалет	too-a-LET
Food	Їжа	YEE-zha
Water	Вода	vo-DA
PROCEDURES & CONSENT		
You need...	Вам потрібно	vam po-TREEB-NO
Injection	Ін'єкція	een-YEK-tsee-ya
Stiches	Шви	sh-VI
Cast	Гіпсова пов'язка	heep-SO-va pov-YAZ-ka
Crutches	Милиці	MI-li-tsee
Perform surgery on the... (See Body Parts List)	Оперувати на...	o-pe-roo-VA-ti na...
The risks are...	Ризики є...	RI-zi-ki ye...
Bleeding	Кровотеча	kro-vo-TE-cha
Infection	Зараження	za-RA-zhen-nya
Scar	Шрам	sh-RAM
Repeat procedure	Повторити процедуру	pov-to-RI-ti pro-tse-DOO-roo

Iodine	Йод	yod
Damage to your…(See Body Parts List)	Пошкодження…	posh-KO-jen-nya…
Sign here	Підпишіть тут	peed-pi-SHEET toot
TESTS		
X-ray	Рентґенограма	rent-gen-o-HRA-ma
C.A.T. Scan	Комп'ютерна томографія (К.Т.)	kom-P-YOOT-ter-na to-mo-HRA-fee-ya (ka-te)
Ultrasound	Ультразвук	ool-tra-z-VOOK
Catheterization/ bladder catheter	Катетеризація / Катетер / катетер в міхурі	ka-te-ter-ri-ZA-tsee-ya / ka-TE-ter v mee-KHOO-ree
Colonoscopy (from below)/ Endoscopy (from above)	Колоноскопія	ko-lo-no-SKO-pee-ya
Endoscopy	Ендоскопія	en-do-SKO-pee-ya
END OF LIFE		
Do you want us to…	Чи ви хочете щоб ми…	chi vi KHO-che-te sh-CHOB mi…
Perform CPR	Робили Серцево-легеневе оживлення (СЛО)	ro-BI-li SER-tse-vo-le-he-NE-ve o-ZHIV-len-nya (es-el-O)
Defibrillate	Робили дефібриляцію	ro-BI-li de-fee-bri-L-YA-tsee-yoo
Intubate	Інтубувати / Увесли трубу в гортань	een-too-boo-VA-ti / oo-VES-li TROO-boo v hor-TAN
He/she is dead	Він(he) помер / Вона (she) померла	veen (he) po-MER / vo-NA (she) po-MER-la

(cont.)

We did all we could	Ми зробили все, що могли	mi z-ro-BI-li v-se, sh-CHO MO-H-li
DISCHARGE		
You have…(See Medical Prob List)	Ви маєте…	vi MA-ye-te…
He/she is going to stay in the hospital	Він (he)/вона (she) залишається в лікарні	veen (he)/vo-NA (she) za-li-SHA-yet-s-ya v lee-kar-nee
Take "X" pills "Y" times a day for "Z" days	Приймайте "X" пілюлі "Y" рази на день на "Z" днів	pree-MAY-te "X" pee-L-YOO-lee "Y" ra-ZI na den na "Z" d-NEEW
Pills	Пілюлі	pee-L-YOO-lee
Antibiotics	Антибіотики	an-ti-bee-O-ti-ki
Before/after meals	Перед їжою / після їжи	PE-red YEE-zho-yoo / PEES-l-ya YEE-zhi
Return to the ER if…	Повернутися в відділення скорої допомогі якщо…	po-ver-NOO-ti-sya v veed-DEE-len-nya SKO-ro-yee do-po-MO-hi yak-SH-CHO…
Follow up at "X" on "Y"	Ідіть до "X" в "Y"	ee-DEET do "X" v "Y"
You're welcome	Нема за що	ne-MA ZA sh-CHO
Goodbye	До побачення	do-po-BA-chen-nya
MEDICAL PROBS		
AIDS/HIV	СНІД / ВІЛ	sneed (es-en-ee-de) / veel (ve-ee- el)
Anemia	Анемія	a-NE-mee-ya
Arrhythmia	Аритмія	a-RIT-mee-ya
Arthritis	Артрит	ar-TRIT
Asthma	Астма	AST-ma

Bronchitis	бронхіт	bron-KHEET
Cancer	Рак	rak
Cirrhosis	цироз	tsi-ROZ
Cholesterol	холестерол	kho-les-te-ROL
Cold	Простуда	pro-STOO-da
Constipation	Запор (утруднене випорожнення кишок)	ZA-por (oo-TROO-de-ne vi-po-ro-ZHEN-nya ki-shok)
Cyst	Кіста / Циста	KEES-ta / TSIS-ta
Diabetes	Діябет	dee-ya-BET
Dialysis	Діяліза	dee-ya-LEE-za
Diverticulitis	Дивертикуліт	di-ver-ti-koo-LEET
Emphysema	Емфізема	em-fee-ZE-ma
Fibroids	Фіброма	fee-BRO-ma
Fracture	Перелом	pe-re-LOM
Flu	Грип	Hrip
Gallstones	Жовчний камінь	ZHOV-ch-nee KA-meen
Gastritis/GERD	Гастрит / Піроз	has-TRIT / pee-ROZ
Hepatitis	Гепатит / запалення печінки	he-pa-TIT / za-PA-len-nya pe-CHEEN-ki
Heart attack	Інфаркт / Удар серця	een-FARKT / oo-DAR SER-ts-ya
Heart disease	Серцева хвороба	ser-TSE-va kh-vo-RO-ba
Heart failure	Параліч (провал) серця	pa-RA-leech (PRO-val) SER-ts-ya
Hypertension	Підвищений кров'яний тиск	peed-VISH-che-niy krov-YA-niy tisk

(cont.)

Indigestion	Нетравлення	nev-TRAV-len-nya
Kidney stone	Галька / нирковий камінь	HAL-ka / nir-KO-viy KA-meen
Lupus	Вовчак	vov-CHAK
Migraine	Мігрень	mee-HREN
Murmur	Шепіт / Шум	she-PEET / shoom
Pacemaker	Стимулятор серця (Синусний вузол серця)	sti-moo-L-YA-tor SER-ts-ya (SI-noos-nee VOO-zol SER-ts-ya)
Pneumonia	Пневмонія / запалення легенів	p-new-MO-nee-ya / za-PA-len-nya le-HE-neew
Seizures	Апоплексичний удар	a-po-plek-SICH-nee oo-DAR
STD	Статева хвороба	sta-TE-va kh-vo-RO-ba
Stroke	Удар мозку	oo-DAR MOZ-koo
Ulcer	Виразка	VI-raz-ka
Ulcerative colitis	Виразковий коліт	vi-raz-KO-vee ko-LEET
UTI	Захворювання сечових шляхів	za-kh-vor-yoo-VAN-nya se-cho-VIKH sh-l-ya-KHEEW
BODY PARTS		
Abdomen	Живіт	zhi-VEET
Ankle	Кісточка / щиколотка	KEES-toch-ka / SH-CHI-ko-lot-ka
Appendix	Апендикс/ червоподібний відросток	a-PEN-diks/ cher-vo-po-DEEB-nee veed-RO-stok
Arm	Рука	roo-KA
Artery	Артерія	ar-TE-ree-ya

Back	Спина	spi-NA
Bladder	Міхур	mee-KHOOR
Blood	Кров	krov
Bone	Кість	keest
Brain	Мозок	MO-zok
Breast	грудь	hrood
Calf	Литка	LIT-ka
Chest	Груди	HROO-di
Chin	Підборіддя	peed-bo-REED-d-ya
Ear	Вухо	VOO-kho
Elbow	Лікоть	LEE-kot
Eye	Око	O-ko
Face	Лице / обличчя	li-TSE / ob-LICH-ch-ya
Finger	Палець	PA-lets
Foot	Нога	no-HA
Hand	Рука	roo-KA
Head	Голова	ho-lo-VA
Heart	Серце	SER-tse
Gallbladder	Жовчний міхур	ZHOV-ch-niy MEE-khoor
Jaw	Щелепа	sh-che-LE-pa
Joint	Суглоб	soo-h-LOB
Kidney	Нирка	NIR-ka
Knee	Коліно	ko-LEE-no
Leg	Нога	no-HA
Liver	Печінка	pe-CHEEN-ka

(cont.)

Mouth	Рот	rot
Muscle	М'яз	m-yaz
Neck	Шия	SHI-ya
Nerve	Нерв	nerv
Nose	Ніс	nees
Ovary	Яєчник	Ya-YECH-nik
Pancreas	Панкреас / Підшлункова залоза	PAN-kre-as / peed-sh-loon-KO-va za-LO-za
Penis	Пеніс / статевий член	PE-nees / sta-TE-viy ch-LEN
Prostate	Простата / передміхурова залоза	PRO-sta-ta / pe-red-mee-khoo-RO-va za-LO-za
Rectum	Пряма кишка	p-r-YA-ma KISH-ka
Rib	Ребро	reb-RO
Shoulder	Плече	PLE-che
Skin	Шкіра	sh-KEE-ra
Spleen	Селезінка	se-le-ZEEN-ka
Spine	Хребет	kh-re-BET
Stomach	Шлунок	sh-LOO-nok
Teeth	Зуби	ZOO-bi
Testicle	Яєчко	ya-YECH-ko
Throat	Горло	HOR-lo
Thyroid	Щитовидна залоза	sh-chi-to-VID-na za-LO-za
Toe	Палець на нозі	PA-lets na NO-zee
Tonsils	Тонзил / Мигдалеподібна залоза	TON-zil / mi-h-da-le-po-DEEB-na za-LO-za

Tongue	Язик	ya-ZIK
Uterus	Матка	MAT-ka
Vagina	Вагіна / Піхва	VA-hee-na / PEEKH-va
Vein	Жила	ZHI-la
Wrist	Зап'ясток	ZA-p-ya-stok

NUMBERS

How many (times)?	Скільки (разів)?	SKEEL-ki (ra-ZEEW)?
0	Нуль	Nool
1	Один	o-DIN
2	Два	d-va
3	Три	tri
4	Чотири	cho-TI-ri
5	П'ять	P-YAT
6	Шість	sheest
7	Сім	seem
8	Вісім	VEE-seem
9	Дев'ять	DEV-yat
10	Десять	DES-yat
11	Одинадцять	o-di-NAD-ts-yat
20	Двадцять	d-VAD-ts-yat
30	Тридцять	TRID-ts-yat
40	Сорок	SO-rok
50	П'ятдесят	p-yat-des-YAT
60	Шістдесят	sheest-des-YAT
70	Сімдесят	seem-des-YAT

(cont.)

80	Вісімдесят	vee-seem-des-YAT
90	Дев'яносто	Dev-ya-NO-sto
100	Сто	Sto

Vietnamese—Tiếng Việt

WORD/PHRASE	TRANSLATION	ENGLISH PRONUNCIATION
Vietnamese	Tiếng Việt	tee-en vee-et
INTRODUCTION & REGISTRATION		
Hello	Xin chào	sin JAU
I am a doctor / nurse *(add your name)*	Tôi tên [là bác sĩ] *(doctor)* / [y tá] *(nurse) (add your name)*	toy tey-n [la bak si = doctor] / [ee ta = nurse] *(add your name)*
What is your name?	Tên của [ông / bà / bạn] *(addressing: Mr./Mrs./a young person respectively)* là gì ?	tey-n koo-a [ang/ba/bạn] *(addressing: Mr./Mrs./a young person respectively)* la zee ?
Who is your doctor?	Bác sĩ của [ông / bà / bạn] *(addressing: Mr./Mrs./a young person respectively)* là ai ?	bak see koo-a [ang/ba/bạn] *(addressing: Mr./Mrs./a young person respectively)* la ay
How old are you?	[Ông / bà / bạn] *(addressing: Mr./Mrs./a young person respectively)* bao nhiêu tuổi ?	[ang/ba/bạn] *(addressing: Mr./Mrs./a young person respectively)* bau nyee-oo too-ee?
Birthdate?	Ngày sinh ?	n-gay sing?
Telephone number?	Số điện thoại ?	so dee-in to-ay?
Address?	Địa chỉ ?	dee-a chee?
Social security number?	Số an ninh xã hội ?	so ang nin sa hoy?
Insurance?	Bảo hiểm sức khoẻ ?	bau hi-eem suk kho-e?

(cont.)

BASICS		
Do you understand?	Ông / bà / bạn có hiểu không ?	ang/ba/ban ko hee-oo k-hong?
Yes	Đúng or Vâng	doo-ng or vang
No	Sai	say
Please	Làm ơn	lam u-n
Thank you	Cám ơn	kam u-n
Sorry	Xin lỗi	sin loy
I don't understand	Tôi không hiểu	toy k-hong hee-oo
Repeat	Lập lại	lap lay
Speak slowly	Nói chậm lại	noy k-ham lay
Answer "yes" or "no"	Trả lời "đúng" hay "sai"	tra loy "doo-ng" hay "say"
Here	Đây	dey
This	Cái này	kai ney
It's alright (consoling)	Không sao đâu	k-hong sau dau
I'll be right back	Tôi sẽ quay trở lại	toy se wey tro lay
GENERAL		
What's wrong?	Chuyện gì xảy ra ?	choo-en zhee sey ra?
Pain	Đau	dau
Do you have pain?	Ông / bà có đau không ?	ang/ba ko dau k-hong?
Does the pain radiate?	Cơn đau có lan đi không ?	kon dau ko lan dee k-hong?
Where (show me)	Ở đâu (chỉ cho tôi) ?	U dau (c-hee c-ho toy)?
Gone now	Hết rồi	h-et roy
Still present	Vẫn còn	van kon

Sudden/gradual onset	Đột ngột / từ từ	dot n-got / tu tu
What bothers you the most?	Chuyện gì làm ông/bà khó chịu nhất ?	choo-en zhee lam ang/ba k-ho chee-oo n-hat?
Why did you come today?	Tại sao ông/bà đến hôm nay ?	tay sau ang/ba deyn hom ney?
QUALITY		
If '0' is no pain and 10 is maximum pain, what number do you have now?	Nếu 'không' là không đau và mười là đau nhất, [ông = speaking to man/ bà = speaking to a woman] ở mức độ nào	ne-oo "k-hong" la k-hong dau va mu-ee la dau n-hat, [ang = speaking to a man / ba = speaking to a woman] o muk do nau
Burning	Nóng rát	no-ong rat
Constant	Kéo dài	keo zay
Dull	Âm ỉ	am ee
Intermittent	Từng cơn	tung ku-n
Pressure	Sức đè	suk de
Severe	Dữ dội	zhu zhoy
Sharp/prickly pains	Buốt/Nhói	bu-ot / Nho-oi
Throbbing	Đập mạnh	da-ap man
ASSOCIATED SYMPTOMS		
Onset during… (before/after)	Triệu chứng bắt đầu … (trước / sau)	tree-oo c-hung bæt dau … (tru-ot / sau)
Worse (with…)	Tệ hơn (với …)	te hon (voy ….)
Better (with…)	Đỡ hơn (với ….)	du hon (voy ….)
Cough	Ho	ho

(cont.)

Deep breath	Hít thở sâu	h-eet tu so-u
Emotional upset	Chuyện buồn	choo-en bu-oon
Food	Đồ ăn	do æn
Movement	Chuyển động	choo-en do-ong
Nothing	Không gì	k-hong zee
Positioning	Vị trí	vee tree
Rest	Nghỉ ngơi	n-gee n-goy
Walking	Đi bộ	dee bo
TIME COURSE		
For how long?	Trong bao lâu ?	trong bau lau?
Today	Hôm nay	hom ney
Yesterday	Hôm qua	hom wa
How many...	Có bao nhiêu....	ko bau n-hee-oo....
Months/weeks/days/hours/seconds	Tháng / Tuần / Ngày / Giờ / Giây	tang / too-an / ngey/ zho / zhey
Still present?	Vẫn còn	van kon
Gone now?	Hết rồi	het roy
How long did it last? (See Numbers List)	Nó xảy ra bao lâu ?	no sey ra bau lau?
Have you had this before?	Ông / bà có triệu chứng này bao giờ chưa ?	ang/ ba ko tree-oo c-hung ney bau zu c-hua?
How many times?	Bao nhiêu lần rồi ?	bau n-hee-oo lan roy?
When was the last time?	Lần cuối khi nào ?	lan koo-oy khee nau?
New	Mới	moy
Old	Cũ	koo

CONTEXT		
Did you…?	Có phải ông / bà … ?	ko fay ang / ba….?
fall	Té	te
trip	Trượt té	tru-ot te
faint	Xỉu	see-oo
twist	trật chân	trak chan
get hit	Bị đánh	bee dan
get burned	Bị phỏng	bee pho-ong
get assaulted	Bị hành hung	bee han hoo-ng
get bitten (human/dog/cat/insect)	Bị cắn	bee kan
PAST MEDICAL HISTORY		
Take medication?	Có uống thuốc không ?	ko oo-ong thoo-ok k-hong?
(aspirin/antibiotics)	Aspirin / thuốc kháng sinh	Aspirin / thoo-ok k-hang sin
Do you have (See also Medical Problem List)…	Ông / bà có…(Xem các căn bệnh)	ang / ba ko…
allergies	Dị ứng	zee ung
medical problems	Các căn bệnh	ca-ac ca-an ben
Do you have problems of the…(see Body Parts List)	Ông có vấn đề của…(đọc phần bộ phận thân thể)	ang ko van dey koo-a…(doc fan bo fan t-han t-he)
SURGICAL HISTORY		
Have you had surgery?	Ông / bà có mổ bao giờ chưa ?	ang / ba ko mo bau zho c-hua?

(cont.)

Surgery on/"to remove"…(see Body Parts List)	Mổ ở ….(Xem bộ phận cơ thể)	mo u…..
SOCIAL HISTORY		
Smoke?	Hút thuốc ?	hoot t-hoo-ok?
Drink?	Uống rượu ?	oo-ong ru-oo ?
Take drugs?	Có dùng Ma túy ?	Co zung ma too-ee?
Recent travel?	Du lịch thời gian gần đây?	zoo leet t-hoy zan gun dey?
Are you sexually active?	Bạn đang hoạt động tình dục ?	ban dan ho-at dong tee-n zhoo-c?
Do you use condoms?	Bạn có dùng bao cao su ?	ban ko zoo-ung bau kau su?
Homosexual	Đồng tính	dong teen
SYSTEMS REVIEW		
Do you have…	Bạn có …. ?	Ban ko….?
GENERAL		
Fever	Sốt	sot
Chills	Lạnh	lan
Weight loss	Sụt cân	soo-t kan
Fatigue	Mệt mỏi	meyt moy
Sick contact	Gần người bệnh	gun n-gu-ee bey-n
HEENT		
Sore throat	Đau cổ họng	dau ko hong
Runny nose	Chảy nước mũi	chey nu-oc moo-ee
Nosebleed	Chảy máu mũi	chey mau moo-ee
Ear pain	Đau lỗ tai	dau lo tay
Ear ringing	Ù tai	U tay

Decreased hearing	Nghe không rõ	n-ge k-hong ro
EYE		
Eye pain	Đau mắt	dau mæt
Blurry vision	Nhìn không rõ	n-hee-n k-hong ro
Diplopia	Thấy hai vật	t-hey hay vat
Foreign body sensation	Cảm thấy cơ thể khác lạ	kam t-hey co the kha-ac la
Contact lenses	Kính sát tròng	kin sat trong
CARDIAC		
Chest pain	Đau ngực	dau n-guk
Palpitations	đánh trống ngực	dan trong n-guk
Orthopnea	Khó thở khi nằm	kho t-hu khee næm
Dyspnea on exertion	Khó thở khi hoạt động	kho t-hu khee ho-at dong
Fainting (syncope)	Xỉu	see-oo
Leg swelling	Sưng chân	sung c-han
How many pillows?	Bao nhiêu gối ?	bau n-hee-oo goy?
PULMONARY		
Trouble breathing	Khó thở	kho t-hu
SOB	thở nông	t-hu nong
Cough	Ho	ho
Sputum	Đờm	du-m
Pain on inspiration	Đau ngực khi hít thở	dau n-guk khee h-eet t-hu?
Hemoptysis	Ho ra máu	ho ra mau

(cont.)

GI		
Abdominal pain	Đau bụng	dau bung
Nausea	Buồn nôn	boon non
Vomiting	Nôn	non
Vomiting blood	Nôn ra máu	non ra mau
Coffee ground emesis	Nôn ra màu đỏ bầm	non ra mau do bæm
Anorexia	suy nhược	soo-ee n-hu-oc
Diarrhea	Tiêu chảy	tee-oo c-hey
Difficulty swallowing	Khó nuốt	kho noot
BRBPR	Máu đỏ ở hậu môn	mau do o hau mon
Melena	Phân màu đen	fan mau den
Pain after eating	Đau bụng sau khi ăn	dau bung sau khee æn
Worms	Sán Lãi	Sa-an la-ee
Constipation	Bị bón	bee bon
GU		
Painful urination	Đau khi tiểu	dau khee tee-oo
Urgent urination	mót tiểu	mot tee-oo
Frequent urination	Tiểu thường xuyên	tee-oo t-hu-ong soo-en
Bloody urination	Tiểu ra máu	tee-oo ra mau
Discharge: vaginal/penile	tiết dịch: âm đạo / dương vật	tee-et zhee-t : am dau / zhu-ong vat
PSYCH		
Anxiety	lo âu	lo au
Depression	Trầm cảm	tram kam

Suicidal thoughts	Muốn tự tử	moo-on tu tu
Homicidal thoughts	Muốn giết người	moo-on zhee-et n-gu-ee
Medication overdose	Uống thuốc quá liều	u-ong t-hoo-ok wa lee-oo
Hear voices	Nghe tiếng nói	n-ge tee-eng noi
NEURO		
Headache	Nhức đầu	n-huk dau
Worst headache of life	Đau đầu nhất từ trước đến giờ	dau dau n-hat tu tru-ok deyn zu
Weakness	Yếu	ee-oo
Dizzy	Chóng mặt	chong mæt
What is your name?	Tên bạn là gì ?	teyn ban la zee?
Where are we?	Chúng ta đang ở đâu ?	choo-ng ta dang u dau?
What is the year/month/date?	Bây giờ năm / tháng / ngày nào ?	bey zu næm / t-hang / ngey nau?
Bowel dysfunction	Rối loạn tiêu hóa	ro-ee lo-an tee-oo ho-a
Bladder dysfunction	Rối loạn tiết niệu	ro-ee lo-an tee-et nee-oo
Photophobia	Sợ ánh sáng	su an sang
Tingling/numbness	Tê / mất cảm giác	te / mat kam zhak
Decreased strength in… (See Body Parts List)	Giảm sức mạnh ở….	zam suk man u…..
Seizure	Co giật	ko zat
Difficulty walking	Đi khó khăn	dee kho khæn

(cont.)

Difficulty speaking	Nói khó khăn	noy kho khæn
Spinning (vertigo)	Chóng mặt (quay cuồng)	chong mæt (qua-ee kuo-ong)
Confusion	nhầm lẫn	n-ham lan
MISC		
Lump	U	oo
Itching	ngứa	n-gua
Bruising	Bầm	bam
Rash	Sởi	so-ee
Swelling	Sưng	sung
Jaundice (yellow skin)	Vàng vọt	vang vot
GYNECOLOGIC		
Vaginal bleeding	Chảy máu âm đạo	chey mau am dau
Heavy	Nhiều	n-hee-oo
Irregular	Không đều	khong de-oo
Absent	Không có	khong ko
Vaginal discharge	Âm đạo tiết dịch	am dau tee-et zheet
Pelvic pain	Đau xương chậu	dau xu-ong cha-ou
Rape	Hãm hiếp	ham heep
Pain with intercourse	Đau khi làm tình	dau khee lam tin
Contraceptive	Dụng cụ tránh thai	zhung ku tran t-ha-ee
OBSTETRIC		
Are you pregnant?	Bạn có thai không ?	ban ko t-ha-ee khong?

LMP how many days ago?	Lần kinh nguyệt vừa rồi cách đây mấy ngày ?	lan k-een n-goo-et vu-a ro-ee k-at dey mey n-gey?
Times pregnant?	Có thai bao nhiêu lần ?	ko t-ha-ee bau n-hee-oo lan?
Times delivered?	Sinh nở bao nhiêu lần ?	seen no bau n-hee-oo lan?
Miscarriage	Sẩy thai	sey t-ha-ee
Abortion	Phá thai	fa t-ha-ee
Fluid leakage	Dung dịch chảy ra	zhung zhee-t chey ra
Contraction	Co thắt	ko t-hæt
Fetal movement	Bào thai chuyển động	bau t-ha-ee c-hoo-en dong
TRAUMA		
How many hours ago did you eat last?	Bạn ăn cách đây mấy giờ ?	ban æn k-at dey mey zho?
Lost consciousness?	bất tỉnh?	but tin?
Tetanus within 5 years?	Ngừa uốn ván trong vòng năm năm ?	n-gua oo-ong van trong vong næm næm?
PEDIATRIC		
How old?	Bao nhiêu tuổi ?	bau n-hee-oo too-ee?
Vaccines up to date?	Vacxin đầy đủ ?	vak-sin dey doo?
Urinating normally	Đi tiểu bình thường	dee tee-oo been t-huong
Taking liquids	Uống nước	oo-ong nu-oc
Increased crying	Khóc nhiều hơn	k-hoc n-hee-oo hu-n
Ingestion	Ăn	æn

(cont.)

Foreign body	Vật lạ (ví dụ : có một vật ở trong con của bạn)	vat la (vee zhoo : ko mok vat o tron kon koo-a ban)
Premature	Đẻ sớm	de som
Birth complications	Đẻ khó	de k-ho
PHYSICAL EXAM/INSTRUCTION		
Sit down (please)	Xin hãy ngồi xuống	seen hey n-goy soo-ong
Lie down	Nằm xuống	næm soo-ong
Come here	Lại đây	lay dey
Relax	Thư dãn	thu - gi-an
Don't move	Đừng di chuyển	dung zhee c-hoo-en
Open your mouth	Hả miệng ra	ha mee-eng ra
Say "ahh"	Nói "ahhhhh"	noy "ahhhhh"
Swallow	Nuốc vào	noo-ok vao
Breath deeply	Thở sâu	t-ho sau
Hold your breath	Ngừng thở	n-gung t-ho
Cough	Ho	ho
Push	Đẩy	dey
Pull	Kéo	keo
Follow my finger	Nhìn ngón tay của tôi	n-heen ngon tey koo-a toy
Close your eyes	Nhắm mắt lại	n-ham mæk lay
Smile	Cười	ku-ee
Can you feel this?	Bạn có cảm giác không ?	ban ko kam zhat khong ?
Copy this (movement)	Bắt chước tôi	bæk k-hu-ot toy

I am going to put a finger in your rectum	Tôi sẽ để một ngón tay vào hậu môn của bạn	toy se dey mot n-gon tey va-o hau mon koo-a ban
I am going to examine your vagina	Tôi sẽ khám âm đạo của bạn	toy se kham am dau koo-a ban

REASSESSMENT

Do you feel better?	Bạn có thấy đỡ hơn không ?	ban ko t-hey du hon k-hong ?
Do you feel worse?	Bạn cảm thấy mệt hơn ?	ban kam t-hey met hon ?

PATIENT WORDS

I hurt	Tôi đau	toy dau
Help!	Cứu !	ku-oo !
Bathroom	Nhà tắm	n-ha taem
Food	Đồ ăn	do aen
Water	Nước uống	nu-oc oo-ong

PROCEDURES & CONSENT

You need...	Bạn cần	ban kan....
Injection	Tiêm	tee-m
Stiches	Muỗi khâu	moo-ee kha-oo
Cast	bó bột	bo bot
Crutches	Cái nạng	ka-ee nan
Perform surgery on the... (See Body Parts List)	Giải phẫu ngay (Xem bộ phận cơ thể)	zha-ee fa-oo n-gey
The risks are...	Những nguy hiểm gồm	n-hung n-goo-ee hee-m gom...
Bleeding	Ra máu	Ra máu
Infection	Nhiễm trùng	n-heem trung

(cont.)

Scar	Theo	t-he-o
Repeat procedure	Mổ lại	mo lay
Iodine	Iot	ee-ot
Damage to your…(See Body Parts List)	Hư hại tới (Xem bộ phận cơ thể)	hu ha-ee toy
Sign here	Ký tên ở đây	kee teyn u dey
TESTS		
X-ray	x - quang	x - wang
C.A.T. Scan	chiếu CAT	k-hee-oo KAT
Ultrasound	siêu âm	see-oo am
Catheterization/ bladder catheter	đặt ống thông/ thông bàng quang	dæk ong thong/ thong bang wang
Colonoscopy (from below)/ Endoscopy (from above)	Soi ruột	soy roo-ot
Endoscopy	Nội soi	no-ee soy
END OF LIFE		
Do you want us to…	Bạn muốn chúng tôi ….	ban moo-on k-hung toy
Perform CPR	Thực hiện hô hấp nhân tạo	t-huk hee-en ho hap n-han tau
Defibrillate	Khử rung tim	Khu ru-ong t-eem
Intubate	Đặt ống thở	dæk ong tu
He/she is dead	Ông/ bà đã tắt thở	ang/ba da tæk tu
We did all we could	Chúng tôi đã cố gắng hết sức	k-hung toy da ko gæng het suk
DISCHARGE		

You have…(See Medical Prob List)	Bạn có …(Xem các căn bệnh)	Ban ko ….
He/she is going to stay in the hospital	Anh / cô ta sẽ ở lại bệnh viện	an / ko ta se u lay beyn vee-en
Take "X" pills "Y" times a day for "Z" days	Uống "X" viên "Y" lần mỗi ngày trong "Z" ngày	oo-ong "X" vee-en "Y" lan moy ngey trong "Z" ngey
Pills	Viên thuốc	vee-en thu-oc
Antibiotics	Kháng sinh	k-hang seen
Before/after meals	Trước / sau bữa ăn	tru-ot / sau bu-a æn
Return to the ER if…	Quay lại phòng cấp cứu nếu ….	wey lay fong kap ku-oo ne-oo ……..
Follow up at "X" on "Y"	Tái khám tại "X" ngày "Y"	tay k-ham ta-ee "X" n-gey "Y"
You're welcome	Không có chi	k-hong ko c-hee
Goodbye	Chào	k-hau
MEDICAL PROBS		
AIDS/HIV	SIDA / HIV	SEE-DA / H-EE-V
Anemia	Thiếu máu	t-hee-oo mau
Arrhythmia	loạn nhịp tim	loo-an n-heep t-eem
Arthritis	Viêm khớp	vee-em k-hop
Asthma	bệnh suyễn	ben soo-en
Bronchitis	Viêm phế quản	vee-em fe wan
Cancer	Ung thư	oong t-hu
Cirrhosis	Sơ gan	su gan
Cholesterol	Mỡ trong máu	mu trong mau
Cold	Cảm	kam

(cont.)

Constipation	Bón	bon
Cyst	U nang	oo nang
Diabetes	Tiểu đường	tee-oo du-ong
Dialysis	Lọc thận	lok t-han
Diverticulitis	viêm túi thừa	vee-em too-ee t-hua
Emphysema	khí phế thủng	k-hee fe t-hung
Fibroids	U sợi	oo soy
Fracture	Gãy	gey
Flu	Cúm	kum
Gallstones	Sỏi mật	soy mat
Gastritis/GERD	viêm dạ dày /	vee-em zha zhey
Hepatitis	Viêm gan	vee-em gan
Heart attack	nhồi máu cơ tim	n-hoy mau ko t-eem
Heart disease	Bệnh tim	ben t-eem
Heart failure	Suy tim	soo-ee t-eem
Hypertension	Cao máu	kau mau
Indigestion	Khó tiêu	k-ho tee-oo
Kidney stone	Sạn thận	san t-han
Lupus	Bệnh luput	ben loo-poot
Migraine	Đau nửa đầu	dau nu-a dau
Murmur	Tiếng tâm	tee-eng tam
Pacemaker	máy tạo nhịp	mey tau n-heep
Pneumonia	Viêm phổi	vee-em foy
Seizures	Kinh phong	keen fong
STD	Bệnh phong tình	ben pho-ong teen
Stroke	Tai biến mạch máu não	tay bee-en ma-ach mow na-o

Ulcer	loét	lo-et
Ulcerative colitis	viêm loét đại tràng	vee-em lo-et day trang
UTI	Nhiễm trùng đường tiểu	n-hee-em trung du-ong tee-oo

BODY PARTS

Abdomen	Bụng	bung
Ankle	Mắt cá	mæk ka
Appendix	Ruột dư	roo-ot zhu
Arm	Tay	tey
Artery	động mạch	dong mat
Back	Lưng	lung
Bladder	Bọng đái	bong dey
Blood	Máu	mau
Bone	Xương	su-on
Brain	Não	nau
Breast	Ngực / Vú	n-guk / voo
Calf	Bắp chuối	bæp c-hoo-oy
Chest	Ngực	n-guk
Chin	Cằm	kam
Ear	Tai	tay
Elbow	Cùi chỏ	koo-ee c-ho
Eye	Mắt	mæk
Face	Mặt	mat
Finger	Ngón tay	ngon tey
Foot	Bàn chân	ban k-han
Hand	Bàn tay	ban tey

(cont.)

Head	Đầu	dau
Heart	Tim	teem
Gallbladder	Túi mật	too-ee mak
Jaw	Quai hàm	way ham
Joint	Khớp xương	k-hop su-ong
Kidney	Thận	t-han
Knee	Đầu gối	dau goy
Leg	Chân	chan
Liver	Gan	gan
Mouth	Miệng	mee-en
Muscle	Bắp thịt (also: Cơ)	bæp t-hee-t (ko)
Neck	Cổ	ko
Nerve	Dây thần kinh	zhey t-han k-een
Nose	Mũi	moo-ee
Ovary	Buồng trứng	boo-ong t-rung
Pancreas	Tuyến tụy	too-en too-ee
Penis	Dương vật	zhu-ong vat
Prostate	Tuyến tiền liệt	too-en tee-en lee-et
Rectum	Hậu môn	hau mon
Rib	Xương sườn	su-ong su-on
Shoulder	Vai	va-ee
Skin	Da	zha
Spleen	Lá lách	la l-at
Spine	Xương sống	su-ong song
Stomach	Bao tử	bau tu
Teeth	Răng	ræn
Testicle	Tinh hoàn	teen ho-an

Throat	Cổ họng	ko hong
Thyroid	Tuyến giáp	too-en zhap
Toe	Ngón chân	ngon c-han
Tonsils	Amidan	a-mee-dan
Tongue	Lưỡi	luo-ee
Uterus	Tử cung	tu kung
Vagina	Âm đạo	am dau
Vein	Tĩnh mạch	teen m-at
Wrist	Cổ tay	ko tey
NUMBERS		
How many (times)?	Bao nhiêu (lần) ?	bau n-hee-oo (lan) ?
0	Không	k-hong
1	Một	mok
2	Hai	ha-ee
3	Ba	ba
4	Bốn	bon
5	Năm	næm
6	Sáu	sau
7	Bảy	bey
8	Tám	tam
9	Chín	cheen
10	Mười	mu-ee
11	Mười một	mu-ee mok
20	Hai mươi	ha-ee mu-ee
30	Ba mươi	ba mu-ee
40	Bốn mươi	bon mu-ee

(cont.)

50	Năm mươi	næm mu-ee
60	Sáu mươi	sau mu-ee
70	Bảy mươi	bey mu-ee
80	Tám mươi	tam mu-ee
90	Chín mươi	cheen mu-ee
100	Một trăm	mok træm

RESOURCES

Computer Translators

Applied Language	http://www.appliedlanguage.com/free_translation.shtml
Babelfish	http://babelfish.yahoo.com/
ForeignWord	http://www.foreignword.com/
Google Translator	http://www.google.com/language_tools
Reverso	http://www.reverso.net/
Stars 21	http://www.stars21.com/
Systran	http://www.systransoft.com/translation
Omniglot	http://www.omniglot.com/links/translation.htm
Your Dictionary	http://www.yourdictionary.com/languages.html
World Lingo	http://www.worldlingo.com/en/products_services/worldlingo_translator.html

Miscellaneous

ATT Healthcare Interpreter Network	http://www.hcin.org
ATT "Your World. Your Language"	1-888-855-0811

(Language-specific directory assistance)

CIA World Fact Book	http://www.cia.gov/library/publications/the-world-factbook/
Embassy.org	http://www.embassy.org

(Contact information for foreign embassies in Washington, D.C.)

International Dialing Codes	http://www.appliedlanguage.com/international_dialing_codes.shtml
U.S. Foreign Consular Offices	http://www.state.gov/s/cpr/rls/

(Contact information for foreign consular offices by country in each U.S. state – local consular offices)

Wish there was an additional phrase included? Have a comment?
We are always seeking to improve. Email your feedback to:
MedTranslation@RossDonaldson.com.

NOTES—ARABIC/العَرَبيّة

NOTES—FARSI/ نابز

NOTES—FRENCH/FRANÇAIS

NOTES—GERMAN/DEUTSCHE

NOTES—HINDI/भाषा

NOTES—ITALIAN/ITALIANO

NOTES—JAPANESE/日本語

NOTES—KOREAN/언어

NOTES—MANDARIN/国语 (國語)

NOTES—POLISH/POLSKI

NOTES—PORTUGUESE/PORTUGUÊS

NOTES—RUSSIAN/РУССКИЙ ЯЗЫК

NOTES—SPANISH/ESPAÑOL